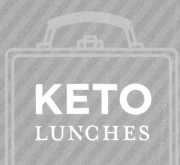

KETO
LUNCHES

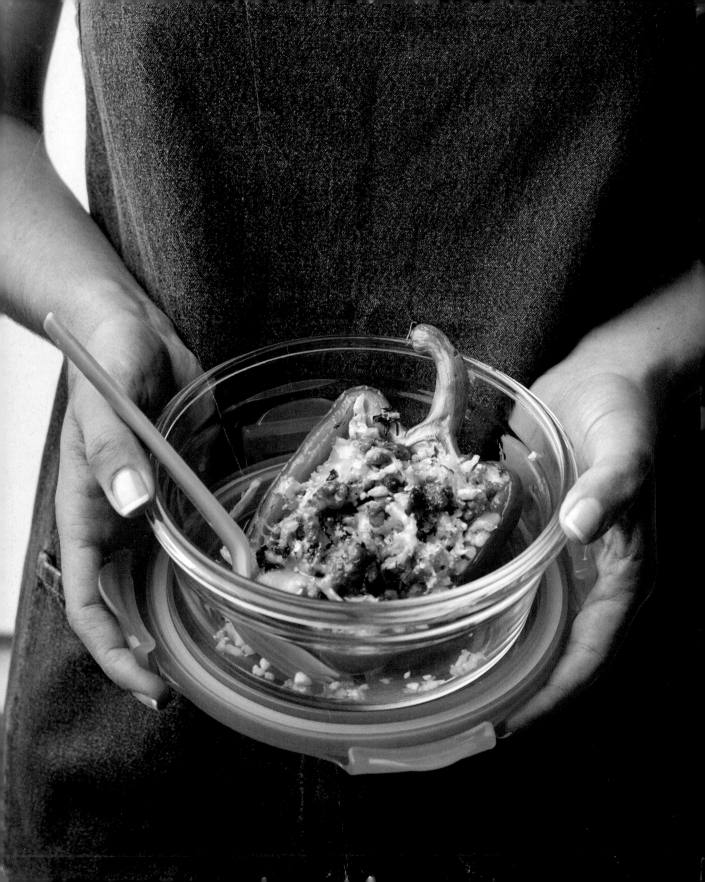

KETO
LUNCHES

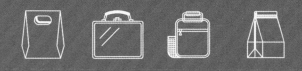

Grab-and-Go,

Make-Ahead Recipes
for High-Power,
Low-Carb
Midday Meals

STEPHANIE PEDERSEN

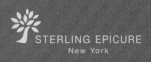

STERLING EPICURE
New York

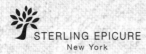

STERLING EPICURE
New York

An Imprint of Sterling Publishing Co., Inc.
1166 Avenue of the Americas
New York, NY 10036

ISBN 978-1-4549-3021-1

Distributed in Canada by Sterling Publishing Co., Inc.
c/o Canadian Manda Group, 664 Annette Street
Toronto, Ontario M6S 2C8, Canada
Distributed in the United Kingdom by GMC Distribution Services
Castle Place, 166 High Street, Lewes, East Sussex BN7 1XU, England
Distributed in Australia by NewSouth Books
45 Beach Street, Coogee, NSW 2034, Australia

For information about custom editions, special sales,
and premium and corporate purchases, please contact
Sterling Special Sales at 800-805-5489 or
specialsales@sterlingpublishing.com.

Manufactured in the United States of America

10 9 8 7 6 5 4 3 2 1

sterlingpublishing.com

Cover design by Jo Obarowski
Interior design by Lorie Pagnozzi
Photography by Bill Milne
(© Sterling Publishing Co., Inc.);
page 35:pingpongcat/Shutterstock.com;
Lunchbox icons /Shutterstock.com

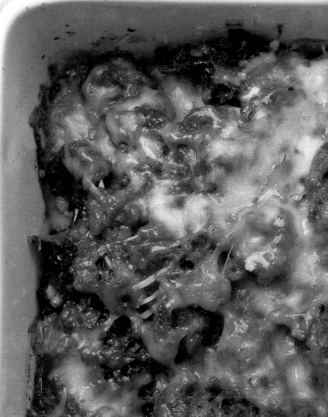

CONTENTS

TITLE PAGE: Keto Italiano Stuffed Peppers (page 103)

Keto Italiano Lasagna (page 124)

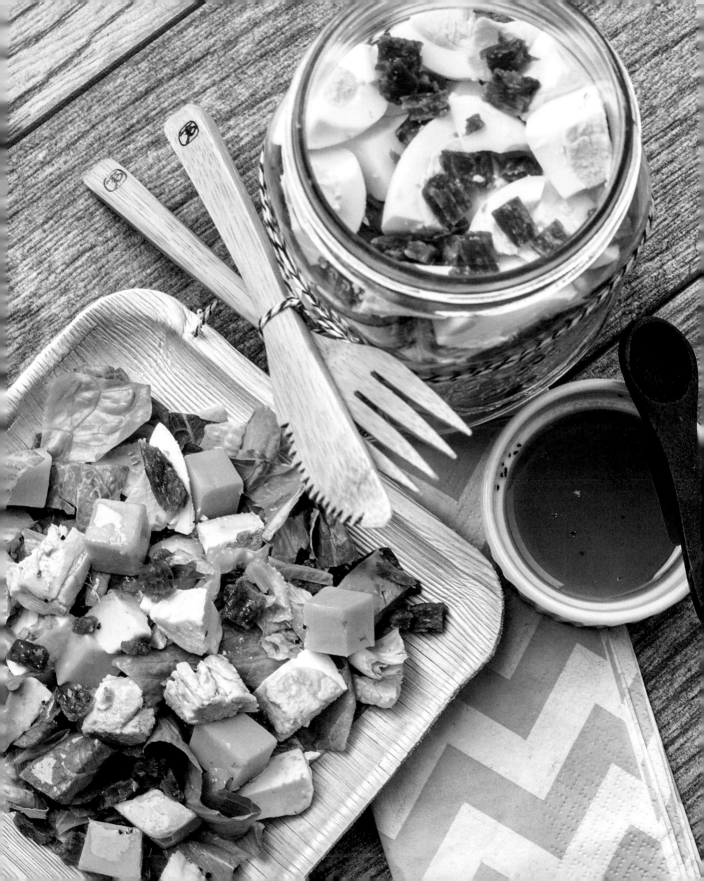

Introduction

> > > > **WHAT IS KETO?** >

Known more formally as "the ketogenic diet," keto eating is one of the hottest health trends. Interestingly, the keto diet is not a new way of eating, neither was it originally intended for weight loss.

Created in the 1920s as a fringe diet to help epileptics, the keto diet has slowly and quietly grown into a diet industry phenomenon. This fat-heavy, carb-shy diet is thought to help heal nervous system disorders (such as epilepsy, seizure disorder, and tic disorder) as well as metabolic disorders (including both type 1 and type 2 diabetes and cardiovascular disease). And although it sounds counterintuitive to expect weight loss while scarfing down large amounts of high-calorie fat, ketogenic eating is said to help eaters slim down, as well.

At the crux of the diet is carbohydrates—specifically, a lack of them. As the theory goes, when you drastically cut down on the amount of carbs you eat, your body begins looking for other sources of energy to help it function. In the absence of carbs, your body's own fat is one of its easiest go-to sources of energy. The process of burning the body's fat for fuel is called ketosis, and it is what the entire ketogenic way of eating is based on. This way of eating encourages your body to use a new fuel source while also causing fewer cravings and less hunger.

< < < < KETO COBB SALAD (PAGE 94)

If that sounds a bit counterintuitive, it is. It is also fat-centric. In fact, in the ketogenic diet endorses 3 or 4 grams of fat for every 1 gram of carbohydrate and protein. This amounts to getting about 75–80 percent of your daily calories from fat. Keto eaters regularly enjoy foods like butter, heavy whipping cream, mayonnaise, bacon, lard, red meat, coconut, avocado, and other fat-heavy foods.

WHY I WROTE *KETO LUNCHES* >

Circling back to lunch: While keto is the hottest diet trend around, it has some specific challenges, the biggest being—yes, you guessed it—lunch! Sure, you can wing it and leave your midday meal to the whims of your office cafeteria, next-door takeout shop, nearby fast food joint, or corner deli. But do that, and chances are you'll cheat or leave without enough food (or the right foods). After all, studies have shown that regardless of what diet you follow, taking the time to make a healthy homemade lunch is one of the surest ways to succeed at losing weight and improving your health.

For keto eaters—who have very specific, non-mainstream eating needs—finding appropriate food is even more challenging, which means that preparing your own keto-specific lunch is one of the surest ways to succeed on the keto diet.

But what to make? And how to find time to make it? *Keto Lunches* has you covered. True, the keto diet has a reputation for being fiddly, time-intensive, and difficult to manage. *Keto Lunches* will teach you how easy it is to make delicious keto-approved lunches that even the busiest of us can find time to throw together. With more than 100 recipes and tons of tips—including shopping advice on how to tackle your biggest keto lunchtime challenges—*Keto Lunches* is an invaluable resource for any keto follower who has ever wondered, "How in the world am I going to manage this thing?" But this book isn't just for keto eaters: Paleo, Atkins, South Beach, and other protein-centric eaters will find that *Keto Lunches* changes their lunchtime life.

After all, most keto followers have a plethora of fantastic, detailed keto bibles that not only offer recipes but also hold readers' collective hand, making it easy to prepare a balanced meals. But this book does something different: It helps keto eaters and carbless dieters create easy, delicious, portable workday lunches. In other words, *Keto Lunches* makes keto doable during the most challenging meal of the day. This book covers something that has been sorely lacking when you consider that there are dozens of keto diet tomes, but none specifically dedicated to very real (and very daunting) challenge of keto-approved workday lunches.

EASIER LUNCH MAKING ﹥﹥﹥﹥﹥﹥﹥﹥﹥﹥﹥﹥﹥﹥﹥﹥﹥﹥﹥﹥﹥﹥﹥﹥﹥﹥

As a a writer, nutrition educator, and mother of three boys, I know what it is like to be so busy that you throw up your hands in despair and turn to premade food. And if that is the direction you ultimately take, please don't feel guilty. It's all good. But because you're reading this book, I've got to believe you'd like some help in creating your own keto-approved lunches. Which is why I am going to offer up these bits of culinary advice to help put lunch-making on automatic:

✱ Practice component cooking. Make a few items (such as Pulled Pork, page 14, and Make-Ahead Chicken Thighs, page 11) that can be used in many recipes or quickly assembled into a delicious keto-approved lunch.

✱ Make items ahead and freeze them. Freezing items in individual portions makes for easy prep during busy nights. Plus, this time-saving tool also helps avoid repetitive meals throughout the week, often a downfall of dieting.

✱ Rely on recipes that offer 2 or 4 servings, so you can eat now *and* later.

✱ Use the time you have. You don't need hours and hours of uninterrupted time in order to make great meals. Instead, get comfy with a few fast, easy, foolproof recipes that you can put together while making dinner the night before or cleaning the kitchen after dinner. (I often cook something while I am doing dishes—in fact, the first two things I usually do before loading the dishwasher each night are to turn on the oven to 350°F and put a pot of salted water on the stove over medium-high heat—just in case I can squeeze in a quick recipe.)

✱ If you like the idea of more relaxed cooking, earmark 2 hours on Saturday or Sunday when you can make large batches of "fatabulous" foods. I personally like to use Saturday mornings for food sourcing and Sunday morning for cooking. Each Saturday, I get up before everyone else and grocery-shop. On Sunday morning, when the kids are all at choir rehearsal, I prep cauliflower and broccoli rice (to cook later), start a pot of chicken or beef or pork stock, and prep some green salad ingredients.

* Use snippets of time when they appear. When I have 10 or 15 unexpected minutes, I will often do some quick meal prep. For me, these include peeling and chopping veggies, defrosting meat or poultry, throwing something in the slow cooker, hopping online to order specialty items, or doing a quick cupboard inventory to see if I am running low on pantry ingredients.

* When you see a sale on a keto-approved ingredient you love, stock up so you have it on hand. Freeze a few salmon steaks or avocados (peel and pit first, rub with oil, then cover with freezer wrap).

* Lunch containers matter. Stock up on single-serve freezer-to-lunch-bag containers (get at least seven). Purchase a heat-insulated container (I like the 12- to 16-ounce sizes). Get a sealable drink cup. Collect a few small containers for sauces

and condiments. Invest in reusable flatware you can keep at your desk. Find a few large, freezerproof containers for big-batch cooking. And don't forget the food wrap! If you love the idea of a cool lunch box or food bag to carry your meal, don't hesitate to buy what you need.

* If you have keto-eating friends or coworkers, double or triple your recipes, divide into single-serve containers, and share. Ask that they do the same. This easy cooking co-op saves huge amounts of time and is a fun way to ensure you all stick to your eating plan.

Recommended equipment to make keto lunch prep even easier:

Food processor

Stand mixer

High-powered blender

Box grater

Spiralizer

2 baking sheets

Large frying pan

Large sauce pot

Mixing bowls

Measuring cups and spoons

Cutting board

Good, sturdy chef's knife.

HAVE FUN!

Humans are hard-wired for fun. If we enjoy something, we stick with it. If something is drudgery, we eventually drop it for other pursuits (and then feel guilty for not being "strong enough" to stick with it).

Hands down, the most important ingredient when it comes to making daily keto lunches is fun. Experiment with recipes, ingredients, best times to be in the kitchen, and more, until you hit upon a groove. Invite your roommate, partner, family, or friends into the kitchen with you. Share meals with coworkers. Pack foods you enjoy eating. And never, ever forget to bring a keto drink with you to work, so you feel loved and pampered. And while you're at it, be sure to slip a decadent fat bomb into your lunch bag—maybe something chocolaty and coconutty like Cocoa-Coconut Balls on page 157. Read on for recipes!

KETO POKE-ISH BOWL (PAGE 86) AND KETO MEATBALLS (PAGE 21) ∨
WITH SPIRALIZED VEGGIE PASTA (PAGE 112) ∨

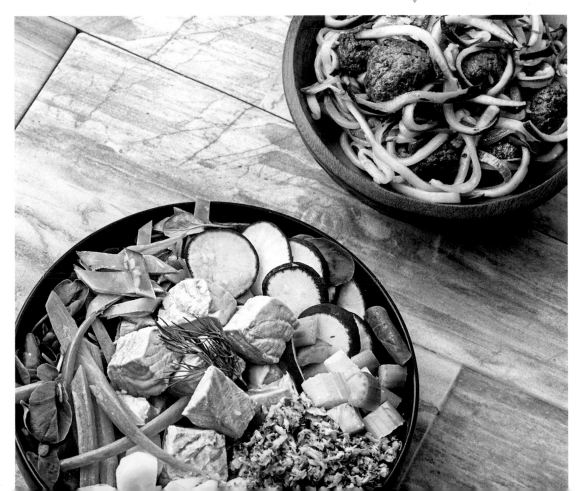

CHAPTER ONE

BUILDING-BLOCK BASICS

If you're like many keto eaters, you may have begun your fat-filled journey with a lot of prepared food. Whether special keto-friendly off-the-shelf (or from-the-freezer) options or prepared delivery services or even keto meal kits, letting someone else do the work makes keto eating easy. But, but, but, . . . outsourcing meal-making is expensive. It also puts you at the mercy of someone else's ingredients. Making your own food not only saves you money but also lets you use your favorite flavors, while avoiding those ingredients that you don't like or that don't agree with you.

Learn the recipes in this chapter and you'll always have something to eat. I like to spend a couple hours over the weekend making these ahead of time, so during a busy week I can truly just grab and go.

THE PERFECT HARD-BOILED EGG

You can use this method to make as many as you'd like, be it just one egg or a dozen. It works on eggs of any size.

8 eggs

1. Place the eggs in a 2-quart saucepan just large enough to contain them without touching each other. Cover them with cool water by 1 inch.

2. Slowly bring the water to a boil over medium heat. When the water has reached a boil, cover the pot and remove it from the heat.

3. For extra large eggs, let sit for 14–16 minutes, depending up on how hard you like the yolk. For large eggs, let sit 10–12 minutes. For medium eggs, let sit 6–8 minutes.

4. Transfer the eggs to a colander in the sink and let cold water run over them to stop the cooking process. You can even plunge the eggs into an ice bath, which some people say makes them easier to peel. Serve immediately or place in a container or egg carton in the refrigerator for up to one week.

PER SERVING: 78 calories, 6g protein, 5g total fat, 1g total carbohydrate

CHICKEN BONE BROTH

This is a great beginner's bone broth recipe, one that will create a lovely chicken broth that can be used as an ingredient or enjoyed alone. To add great flavor depth to the broth, freeze leftover bones from T-bone steaks, pork shoulders, chicken wings, and such in an airtight container and use a variety of bones.

1 (4-pound) chicken, whole, or the carcasses of two or three chickens (parts or whole, such as from a rotisserie chicken)

1 medium onion, peeled and quartered

2 stalks celery, quartered

1 teaspoon whole black peppercorns

1–3 tablespoons salt (Start with 1 tablespoon and adjust with more as needed at the end of cooking.)

OPTIONAL: The green stalk from leeks or scallions (as many as you'd like—even just one—will make your broth more savory; just make sure they are clean), parsley stems, thyme sprigs left whole, fennel fronds, bay leaf

1. Place all ingredients in a large stockpot and cover with about 4 quarts of water, or until all ingredients are covered by about 1 inch.

2. Place the pot over high heat, cover with a lid, and cook until it comes to a rolling boil. Reduce the heat to a simmer and cook for 4 hours. If desired, skim off any fat that collects on the top during the cooking process.

3. After 4 hours, turn off the heat and allow the broth to cool in the pot for 90 minutes or more.

4. Carefully strain out the solids, using a strainer such as a spider or pour the broth into a colander set over a large bowl.

5. Decant the broth into a large container or into individual 1-cup serving containers.

6. Store the broth in the refrigerator for up to three days. If storing longer, freeze it.

PER SERVING (1 CUP): 17 calories, 3g protein, 0g total fat, 1g total carbohydrate

How to clean leeks

If you've ever purchased fresh leeks, you know that dirt often hangs out between the sheathlike leaves. The best way to clean leeks is to chop them (unwashed), place the chopped leeks in a large bowl, and add cold water. Agitate the water with your hands, aggressively moving the chopped leaks around. Wait ten minutes, and all the dirt will have fallen to the bottom of the bowl. Gently lift out the cut leaks (being careful not to disturb the sediment at the bottom of the bowl) with a handheld strainer, slotted spoon, or spider,. Transfer the leeks to a colander and let them drain until dry.

MAKE-AHEAD CHICKEN THIGHS

If you're someone who likes convenience, batch cooking is a lifesaver. Making a batch of these chicken thighs not only ensures something healthy to eat but also gives you a building block for many of the recipes in this book. Go ahead and play with the seasonings if you'd like. If you're not using the finished chicken in another recipe, plan on two thighs per serving.

⅓ cup melted butter, coconut oil, macadamia nut oil, bacon fat, or avocado oil, plus additional for greasing the pan

3–8 garlic cloves, minced

3 tablespoons soy sauce or coconut aminos

Black pepper or red pepper flakes, to taste

½–2 teaspoons fresh rosemary, chives, basil, parsley, thyme, or cilantro, chopped

3½ pounds boneless, skinless chicken thighs

1. Preheat the oven to 425°F.

2. Lightly grease a large baking pan with your fat of choice.

3. In a medium bowl, whisk together the butter, garlic, soy sauce, pepper, and rosemary.

4. Arrange the chicken in the baking pan. Pour the butter mixture over the chicken, coating the pieces thoroughly.

5. Bake the chicken for 25 minutes, then turn the chicken thighs, basting with the pan juices.

6. Return to the oven and bake for an additional 20 minutes or until the juices run clear.

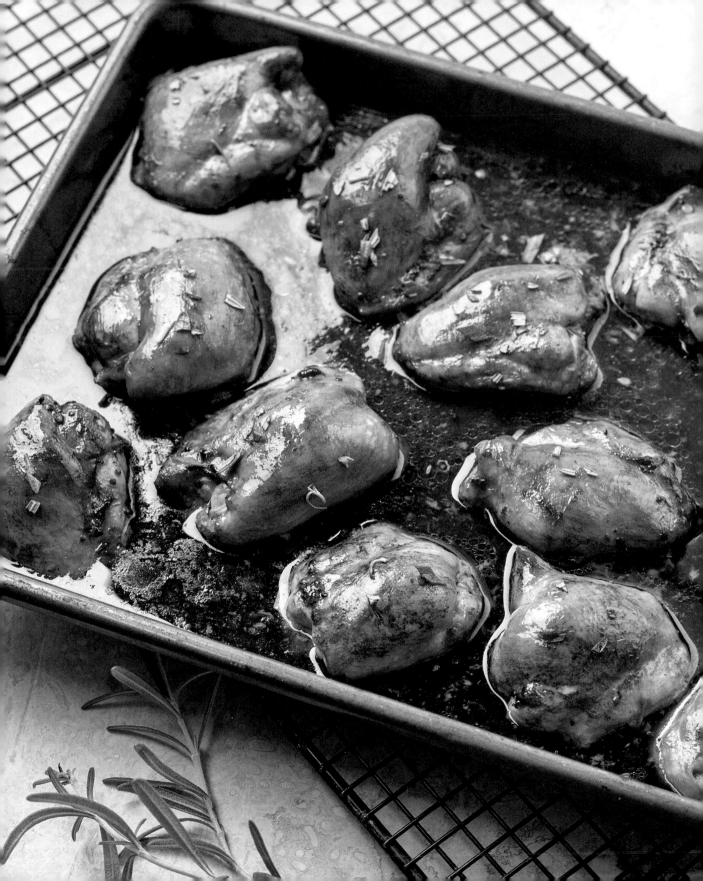

7. Remove the pan from the oven and allow the chicken to cool before placing it in a covered container. Keep in the refrigerator for up to five days.

PER SERVING: 279 calories, 35g protein, 15g total fat, 0g total carbohydrate

* If you do not have soy sauce or coconut aminos in the pantry, replace with 2–3 teaspoons of salt. You can also use different dried spices like cumin or curry powder along with dried herbs, including but not limited to thyme, oregano, parsley, and basil.

PULLED PORK

Pulled pork is not a small-size endeavor, but a slow cooker makes this dish much easier. Pulled pork freezes well and can stay in the freezer for up to three months. Feel free to play with the spices listed here—this recipe is flexible!

1 teaspoon onion powder

1 teaspoon garlic powder

2 teaspoons salt

½ teaspoon black pepper

½ teaspoon paprika

½ teaspoon ground allspice

½ teaspoon celery salt

⅛ teaspoon ground cloves

½ teaspoon mustard powder

¼ cup extra-virgin olive oil, avocado oil, or another oil

¼ cup apple cider vinegar

3 pound boneless pork shoulder or butt, sometimes called picnic roast

OPTIONAL: Keto Barbecue Sauce (page 34)

1. In a small bowl, whisk together all ingredients except the pork and barbecue sauce.

2. Rub the spice mixture all over the pork. Place the pork roast, fat side up, in the slow cooker and cover.

3. Cook on high for 4–6 hours or until the meat is tender and falling apart.

4. Remove the roast to a large bowl and shred using two forks. Discard the melted fat and liquids in the slow cooker, or pour a few tablespoons into the shredded pork for a moister, fattier, pulled pork.

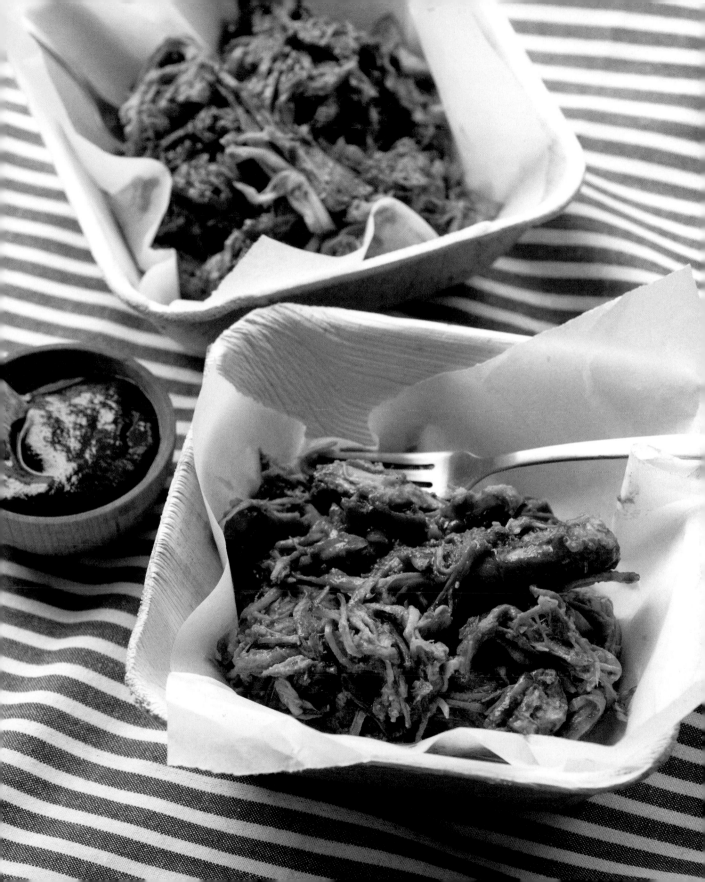

5. Serve as is, or with Keto Barbecue Sauce (page 34).

6. Store in a container in the refrigerator for up to one week.

* Serve the pulled pork as a component of a Keto Bowl (page 88) or as a sandwich on top of Keto Buns (page 42).

PER SERVING: 401 calories, 39g protein, 23g total fat, 0g total carbohydrate

SLOW COOKER COCONUT BEEF ROAST

Makes 4–6 servings

You can start this recipe in the morning and come home to a hot meal—or a meal component that can be used for sandwiches, bowls, tacos, and more.

4 cups beef broth (or Chicken Bone Broth, page 9)

2 large onions, chopped

7 garlic cloves, minced

2 cups sliced mushrooms

1 cup chopped red bell pepper

½ cup sliced celery

Salt and pepper, to taste

½ teaspoon sweet paprika

½ cup canned coconut milk (Do not use "lite.")

2 pound beef rump roast

1. Add the broth, onion, garlic, mushrooms, red pepper, celery, salt and pepper, paprika, and coconut milk to a slow cooker. Stir once.

2. Nestle the roast among the mixture.

3. Put the lid on the slow cooker and cook on low for 6–8 hours or on high for 4–6 hours.

PER SERVING (1 CUP): 275 calories, 29g protein, 16g total fat, 0g total carbohydrate

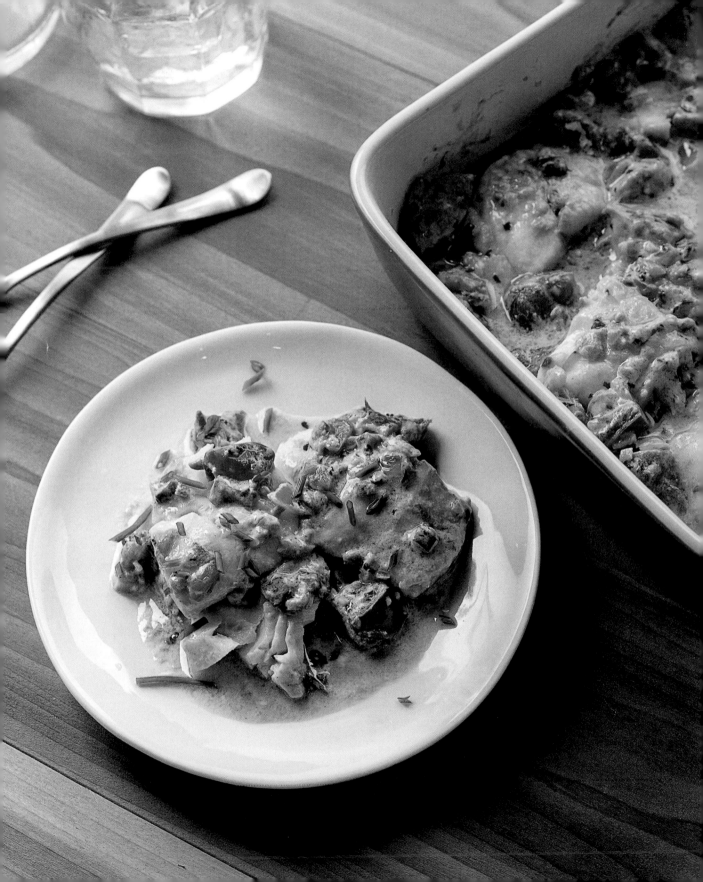

FISH BAKED IN COCONUT MILK

This is an incredibly versatile recipe. Use your favorite mild white fish, such as cod. This recipe also works well with salmon or tuna.

4 teaspoons lemon juice

6 tablespoons liquid coconut oil, divided

1 teaspoon salt, divided

2 pounds thick cod fillets or steaks

2 cups finely chopped onion

2 teaspoons minced garlic

2 teaspoons minced ginger

1 teaspoon minced green Serrano or jalapeño chile pepper

1 cup chopped tomatoes (fresh or drained canned)

5 teaspoons ground coriander

1 teaspoon ground cumin

¼ teaspoon cayenne powder

¼ teaspoon ground black pepper

¼ teaspoon ground turmeric

1 teaspoon dried parsley

½ cup canned coconut milk

OPTIONAL: ¼ cup chopped chives, parsley, or cilantro for garnish

1. Lightly grease a baking dish with coconut oil. Make sure the dish is large enough to hold the fish in a single layer. Set aside.

2. In a small bowl, whisk together the lemon juice, 2 tablespoons of the coconut oil, and ½ teaspoon of the salt. Set aside.

3. Cut the fillets crosswise into 2-inch-wide strips. Pour the lemon juice mixture over the fish, making sure to coat it evenly. Cover the baking dish and refrigerate for 1 hour.

4. In the meantime, heat the remaining 4 tablespoons of coconut oil in a medium frying pan over medium-high heat. Add the onions and fry until the edges are browned.

5. Add the garlic, ginger, and chile pepper, and stir over medium heat for 2 minutes.

6. Add the tomatoes, coriander, cumin, cayenne powder, black pepper, turmeric, parsley, and the remaining salt. Let the sauce simmer, stirring occasionally until the tomato breaks down into a chunky sauce, about 20–30 minutes.

7. Add the coconut milk and simmer about 5 minutes, until the sauce becomes thick. Cover and set aside.

8. Preheat the oven to 350°F. Remove the fish from the refrigerator. Uncover the baking dish and bake the fish for 10 minutes.

9. Remove the fish from the oven, pour the sauce over the fish, cover tightly with foil, and return to the oven for 15–20 minutes or until the fish is opaque.

10. Garnish, if desired, with chopped herbs such as chives.

PER SERVING (MADE WITH COD): 230 calories, 26g protein, 15g total fat, 5g total carbohydrate

* Many people do not make fish at home because they aren't sure how long to cook it. Here's an easy tip: Insert a fork into a piece of fish at a 45° angle at its thickest point. Pretend the fork is the hand on a clock and scoot it 5 minutes to the left or right, then try to pull up some of the fish. If it flakes beautifully, it is done. If it does not flake or looks translucent, it is undercooked (let it cook 5 minutes more and retest).

KETO MEATBALLS

These versatile meatballs are filled with good keto-friendly fats, such as coconut. For a more Asian-style flavor profile, substitute curry powder for the basil and oregano.

1 tablespoon bacon fat or extra-virgin olive oil

½ cup cream or coconut cream

1 teaspoon salt

Black pepper, to taste

1 teaspoon dried basil

½ teaspoon dried oregano

1 pound ground beef, bison, pork, turkey, or chicken, or a combination

¼ cup unsweetened shredded dried coconut

2 or 3 garlic cloves, minced

¼ cup minced shallot, leek, or onion

OPTIONAL: 2 teaspoons seeded and minced fresh jalapeño or Serrano chile or pickled pepperoncini pepper

1. Preheat the oven to 400°F.

2. In a large bowl, gently mix all ingredients.

3. Divide the meat mixture into 10 equal portions, about $1/4$ cup each. Roll each portion into a ball.

4. Place the meatballs on a baking sheet lined with foil or parchment paper, or lightly greased with any type of oil, and place in the oven. Cook for 20 minutes or until browned and no longer pink in the middle.

5. Remove the baking sheet from the oven. Allow the meatballs to cool on the baking sheet. Once cool, store the meatballs in a sealed container in the refrigerator for up to five days.

PER SERVING: 2 beef meatballs: 290 calories, 18g protein, 20g total fat, 4g total carbohydrate

KETO HUMMUS

Hummus is a healthy, easy, portable dip, dressing, spread, and more, except that it is on the carb-heavy side. This version, which uses steamed cauliflower or raw zucchini (you choose) in place of chickpeas, is a great alternative.

4 cups steamed cauliflower florets or peeled and chopped raw zucchini

¾ cups tahini (sesame paste)

½ cup fresh lemon juice

¼ cup extra-virgin olive oil

4 cloves of garlic

Salt and pepper, to taste

1 tablespoon ground cumin

1. Combine all ingredients in a blender and puree until thick and smooth.

2. Taste and adjust seasonings to your preference.

3. Store for up to one week in a covered container in the refrigerator.

PER SERVING (¼ CUP): ¼ cup 130 calories, 2g protein, 14g total fat, 3g total carbohydrate

* Substitute leftover Cauliflower Rice (page 111) for the steamed cauliflower if that's what you have on hand.

Hummus Quick Changes

Hummus lends itself to an amazing array of flavor variations. Here are some of my favorites—simply make the recipe, and drop one of the following add-ins into the blender with the recipe's primary ingredients:

Jalapeño

Add four or five pickled jalapeño slices, chopped—or an entire pickled jalapeño. I also like to toss in 1 tablespoon of chopped cilantro.

Chipotle

Add a half of a chipotle chile canned in adobo sauce, as well as 1–2 teaspoons of the adobo sauce.

Dill and scallion

Toss in a tablespoon of fresh dill and one scallion, chopped (the white and some of the green portions).

Wasabi

Replace the salt with soy sauce and add 1 teaspoon (or more, if you can handle it) of wasabi paste.

KETO SALAD DRESSING

Everyone needs a good basic salad dressing. Enjoy this as is, or add the optional ingredients for additional flavor. You can also use a different type of vinegar or oil, if desired.

1⅓ cups extra virgin olive oil

1 cup balsamic vinegar

1-2 teaspoons salt, to taste

OPTIONAL: 1-2 teaspoons Dijon or another type of mustard

OPTIONAL: ¼-½ teaspoon garlic or onion powder

OPTIONAL: ¼-½ teaspoon dried or powdered herbs or spices, such as basil, thyme, or oregano

1. Combine everything in a quart jar.

2. Screw on the lid and shake well.

3. Store in the refrigerator for up to two months. Shake before using.

PER SERVING (1 TABLESPOON): 75 calories, 0g protein, 8g total fat, 1g total carbohydrate

✳ Mason jars are great ways to make and store dressing.

PERFECT GUACAMOLE

This guacamole recipe is a classic—always delicious, always easy, and always healthy. Eat it as a snack with celery and jicama sticks or as a topping in the Keto Chicken Enchilada Bowl (page 85).

1 large ripe avocado, peeled and pitted

1 small jalapeño, stem and seeds removed, minced (add more or less, to taste)

¼ cup finely chopped red onion

½ tablespoon fresh lime juice

¼ cup fresh cilantro leaves, finely chopped

¼ teaspoon salt

Dash of cumin

1 Roma tomato, cored and chopped

1 tablespoon cilantro leaves, minced

1. Mash together avocado, jalapeño, onion, lime juice, cilantro, salt, and cumin with a fork until well mixed.

2. Gently stir in the tomatoes and cilantro.

3. Tightly cover the bowl with plastic wrap, ensuring the entire top layer of the guacamole touches the plastic. Refrigerate for up to two days before serving.

PER SERVING (½ CUP): 180 calories, 2g protein, 14g total fat, 7g total carbohydrate

VERSATILE MARINARA SAUCE

This easy recipe can be used to dress Spiralized Veggie Pasta (page 112), as a dipping sauce for your favorite finger foods (I recommend the Sausage Puffs, page 131, or Pizza Pockets on page 58), or in recipes (such as Keto Italiano Lasagna, page 124 or Stuffed Cabbage Rolls, page 121).

1 (28-ounce) can crushed tomatoes or tomato puree

¼ teaspoon black pepper

½ teaspoon red pepper flakes

1 teaspoon onion powder

1 teaspoon garlic powder

1 teaspoon dried basil

1 teaspoon dried oregano

1 teaspoon dried parsley

1 teaspoon salt, or to taste

2 tablespoons red wine vinegar

¼ cup extra-virgin olive oil

1. Place all ingredients into a blender and puree until smooth.

2. Taste and adjust spices and salt if necessary.

PER SERVING ½ CUP: 60 calories, 2g protein, 2g total fat, 9g total carbohydrate

* I like to divide the recipe into a few small dressing-size food containers (for when I want a small amount of the sauce as a dip for pizza rolls and other handheld meals) and some one-cup containers. I freeze a few and store the others in the refrigerator so I can grab one when needed.

HOMEMADE MAYO

Store-bought mayos often include sweeteners and other unwanted additions. Homemade mayo is a cinch to whisk together and ensures a fresh and rich taste. Plus, you can personalize it with garlic or onion powder, as well as dried herbs.

1 large egg yolk, free-range or organic

1 teaspoon Dijon mustard (or Easy-Peasy Mustard (page 29)

¾ cup avocado oil or macadamia nut oil

1 tablespoon apple cider vinegar

1 tablespoon lemon juice

Salt and pepper, to taste

OPTIONAL: ¼–½ teaspoon garlic or onion powder

OPTIONAL: ¼–½ teaspoon dried herb of choice

1. Place the egg yolk and the Dijon mustard in the bowl of a food processor and process on low.

2. As the egg and mustard combine, remove the cover from the feed tube and slowly and steadily drizzle in the oil.

3. When the oil is incorporated, slowly drizzle in the vinegar and lemon juice.

4. Pulse in salt, pepper and any optional ingredients. Taste and adjust the seasonings.

5. Scrape into a jar or airtight container, cover, and store in the refrigerator for up to three weeks.

PER SERVING 1 TABLESPOON: 100 calories, 0g protein, 11g total fat, 0g total carbohydrate

* Make sure all ingredients are at room temperature before you begin.

AVOCADO MAYO

I don't love mayo—it's just too rich for my taste. But I adore this yummy, superfood version. If you don't like cilantro, swap in dill or parsley or another herb—even a small garlic clove. Or leave out the herbs altogether. If you don't have lime juice, lemon juice works well, too.

½ cup mayonnaise (or Homemade Mayo (page 27)

1 avocado, peeled and pitted

¼ cup cilantro, chopped

2 teaspoons lime juice

Salt and pepper, to taste

1. Add the mayonnaise, avocado, cilantro, and lime juice to a food processor or blender and blend until smooth.

2. Add salt and pepper to taste.

PER SERVING (¼ CUP): 185 calories, 1g protein, 18g total fat, 5g total carbohydrate

EASY-PEASY MUSTARD

Mustard is so easy to make in a home kitchen that I've always wondered why people purchase it. This is the most basic of mustard recipes. To switch it up, consider tossing in a handful of your favorite herbs, some lemon zest, a shake or two of a beloved spice, or subbing vinegar or wine for the water.

½ cup dried mustard powder

½ cup water, room temperature

Salt, to taste

1. Combine the mustard powder and water in a medium bowl. Whisk together until smooth.

2. Add salt to taste.

3. Allow mustard to sit for 30 minutes before using. Store in a jar in the refrigerator for up to three weeks.

PER SERVING 1 TABLESPOON: 15 calories, 1g protein, 1g total fat, 0g total carbohydrate

EASY-PEASY KETCHUP

Makes about 1½ cups

This no-sugar, low-carb ketchup is not as sweet as commercially prepared products, but it's every bit as tasty! Adjust the spices to your palate if desired.

1 (6-ounce) can tomato paste

2 tablespoons white wine vinegar, apple cider vinegar, or red wine vinegar

¼ teaspoon dry mustard powder

⅓ cup water, room temperature

¼ teaspoon cinnamon

¼ teaspoon salt

Pinch ground cloves

Pinch ground allspice

OPTIONAL: ⅛ teaspoon cayenne pepper

OPTIONAL: pinch black pepper

1. Combine all ingredients in a medium bowl. Whisk together until smooth.

2. Allow the ketchup to sit for 30 minutes to blend the flavors. Taste, and adjust vinegar, spices, and salt.

3. Store the ketchup in an airtight container in the refrigerator for up to three weeks.

PER SERVING 1 TABLESPOON: 10 calories, 0g protein, 0g total fat, 1g total carbohydrate

KETO HOT SAUCE

Many hot sauces contain a bit of sweetener to temper their heat. This homemade version—which is actually super-easy to make— is sweetener-free. Try this with wings or burgers like the Big-O Bacon Burgers (page 47) or Inside-Out Avocado Burger Pockets (page 45).

18 fresh cayenne peppers (ends and stems removed)

1½ cups white vinegar

2 teaspoons garlic, minced

1 teaspoon salt

1 teaspoon garlic powder

1. Place all ingredients in a small saucepan over medium-high heat.

2. When the mixture reaches a boil, lower the heat to medium-low and simmer, uncovered, for 20 minutes

3. Turn off the heat and remove the saucepan from the burner. Let the mixture cool to room temperature. Once cool, transfer the mixture to a blender and process until smooth.

4. Transfer the mixture back to the saucepan and simmer on medium-low for another 15 minutes.

5. Allow to completely cool to room temperature and store in a jar or covered container in the refrigerator for up to two months.

PER SERVING 1 TEASPOON: 2 calories, 0g protein, 0g total fat, 0g total carb

KETO SALSA

Salsa is such a healthy, delicious way to brighten up your meals. This version—which is sweetener-free—is easy to make using ingredients found in your local grocery store.

2 tablespoons lime or lemon juice

2 tablespoons avocado oil

2 cloves garlic, minced

⅓–½ cup cilantro, roughly chopped

Salt and pepper, to taste

1 small sweet onion, such as Vidalia or Walla Walla

2 fresh jalapeño chile peppers, seeds removed, minced

1 (28-ounce) can diced tomatoes, drained (Save the liquid for another recipe.)

1. In a medium bowl, whisk together the lime juice, avocado oil, garlic, cilantro, salt, and pepper.

2. Stir in the onion, jalapeño, and tomatoes.

3. Store in a covered container in the refrigerator for up to one week.

PER SERVING 1 TABLESPOON: 100 calories, 0g protein, 11g total fat, 0g total carbohydrate

* Personalize this salsa by using a different type of chile for more heat or add other spices, like a bit of cumin or oregano.

CHIPOTLE CREAM SAUCE

This delicious sauce is addictive! You'll love it on poultry, meats, and fish; as a sandwich spread; on nachos and tacos; swirled in soups; as a dip; and more.

1 canned chipotle chile in adobo sauce

1–2 teaspoons adobo sauce from canned chipotle

½ cup mayonnaise

⅓ cup sour cream, coconut cream, or plain full-fat yogurt

¼ cup chopped cilantro

¼ teaspoon ground cumin

Salt, to taste

1. Place all ingredients in a blender or food processor and puree until smooth, about 2–3 minutes or until the mixture is nice and creamy.

2. Place in a jar or covered container and refrigerate for up to three weeks.

PER SERVING ¼ CUP: : 170 calories, 1g protein, 15g total fat, 5g total carbohydrate

KETO BARBECUE SAUCE

Store-bought barbecue sauces are loaded with sweeteners (and carbs!), making them poor choices for keto eaters. This easy-to-make recipe is made without sweet ketchup or the stevia that many keto recipes call for. If you must have some sweetness, go ahead and add a few drops of stevia during step 3.

1 tablespoon bacon fat or avocado oil coconut oil, or macadamia nut oil

1 shallot, finely diced

1 or 2 garlic cloves, finely diced

1 (6-ounce) can tomato paste

¼ cup Easy-Peasy Mustard (page 29), Dijon mustard, or brown mustard

1½ cups water or Chicken Bone Broth (page 9)

1 tablespoon apple cider vinegar

2 teaspoons salt

1 tablespoon chili powder

½ tablespoon smoked paprika

½ teaspoon black pepper

1 teaspoon cumin

¼ teaspoon thyme

1. Heat the fat in a sauté pan over medium-high heat. Add the shallot and garlic and sauté until the shallots are translucent.

2. Add all remaining ingredients, stir well, and let simmer for 5 minutes.

3. Puree in a blender or food processor until smooth.

4. Store in a jar or covered container in the refrigerator for up to one month.

PER SERVING 1 TABLESPOON: 22 calories, 1g protein, 3g total fat, 0g total carbohydrate

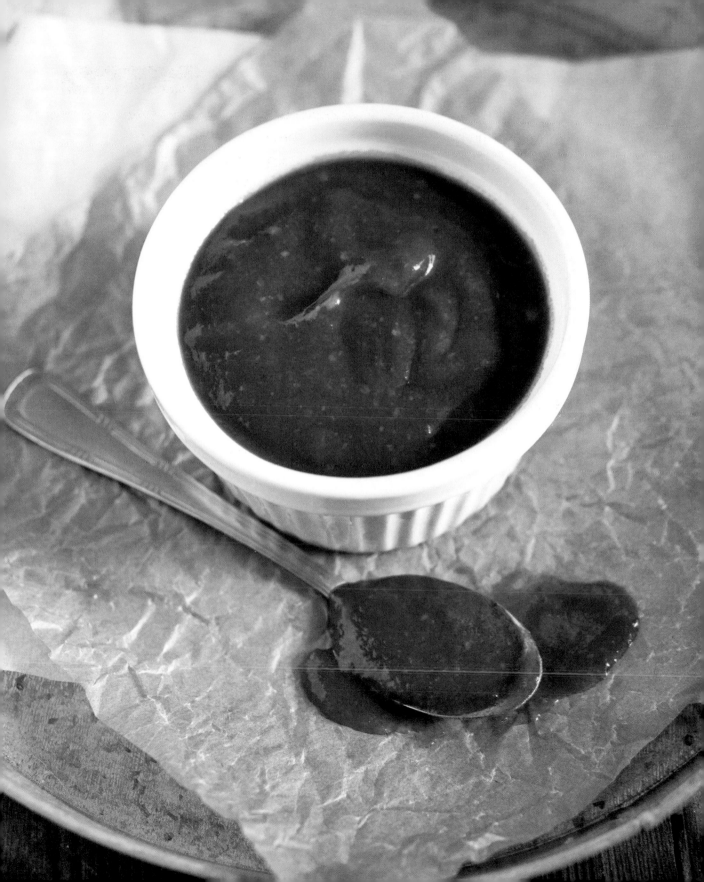

CHAPTER TWO

Wraps, Fatwiches, and Other Handheld Meals

When you hear the words *brown bag lunch,* I bet you think of sandwiches. Maybe tuna on rye or a chicken wrap, or roast beef on a roll, even a stromboli. For us keto eaters, however, sandwiches of any kind are tricky: Bread (even whole-grain bread or gluten-free bread), wraps, and rolls are incredibly high in carbs. The good news is we keto eaters can enjoy sandwiches—they just don't look quite like the sandwiches most of us grew up with. Fortunately they are just as delicious as traditional sandwiches, as the recipes in this chapter prove.

Keto Wraps

Here are a few easy wrap recipes to play with. Fill with whatever keto-friendly fillings you'd like!

ICEBERG WRAPS

Makes varying amounts

Iceberg lettuce is the butt of many culinary jokes. True, it's mostly water and some fiber, but wow, does it make an excellent keto sandwich wrapper. As hardy as iceberg is, however, it can be a bit fiddly in the wrap department. Here is a quick rundown on how to use the leaves:

1. Choose a head that is large and unblemished; its leaves will be the best.

2. Without cutting into the lettuce leaves, remove the core at the base of the head. You can do this by turning the head of lettuce upside down and carving the core out from the bottom of the head. You can then simply pull the core out from the intact head.

3. If there are any withered or torn leaves on the outside of the head, gently remove those, as well.

4. Fill large mixing bowl or pot with cold water. Gently submerge the head of lettuce, holding it under the water if it floats up. Your goal is to get water between the layers of leaves. This helps separate them in a way that keeps the leaves large and tear-free. (You can also do this by simply turning your faucet on and allowing water to run into and through the lettuce.)

5. While the lettuce is underwater, gently remove the leaves, stacking them in a waiting colander or laying them flat on a clean dishtowel.

6. To use as a wrap, place the filling in the lower third of the leaf, fold in the sides, then roll the same way you'd roll a burrito.

7. Unused leaves can be stacked between dry paper towels.

PER SERVING: 2 calories, 0g protein, 0g total fat, 1g total carbohydrate

PALEO-STYLE KETO WRAP

Makes 4 wraps

I got this recipe from a paleo-loving friend. It uses coconut flour and ground psyllium husks (you can whir psyllium husk in your coffee grinder) to make a puffy, soft, low-carb wrap. I find they are easier to fill and wrap when they are warm or room temperature. Play with the spices to make flavored wraps.

½ cup coconut flour

2 tablespoons ground psyllium husks

½ teaspoon salt

¼ cup coconut oil

1 cup boiling water

OPTIONAL: ¼–½ teaspoon onion or garlic powder

OPTIONAL: ½ teaspoon dried basil, oregano, chili powder, curry powder, or any other spice or spice mix you enjoy

1. Preheat the oven to 350°F.

2. Lightly grease a sheet of parchment paper (the size of a baking sheet) with coconut oil. Set aside.

3. In the bowl of a stand mixer, whisk together the coconut flour, ground psyllium, salt, and any optional spices.

4. Add the coconut oil and mix on low just until combined.

5. With the mixer on, slowly pour in the hot water. Continue mixing until the dough is smooth and well-combined

6. Cover the mixing bowl with plastic or foil and place in the refrigerator for 15 minutes to cool.

7. Remove the mixing bowl from refrigerator and divide dough into four balls. Place the balls of dough on the greased parchment, leaving a lot of space between each.

8. Using a rolling pin, roll each ball into a circle between ⅛ and ¼ inch thick.

9. Lift the parchment onto a baking sheet and bake for 18–20 minutes.

10. Remove and let cool for 15 minutes before removing each wrap with a spatula. Store unused wraps in the refrigerator for up to two days.

PER SERVING: 130 calories, 2g protein, 11g total fat, 2g total carbohydrate

OMELET WRAP

Makes about 6 (8-inch) wraps

Here's another coconut-based wrap, this one made with mostly eggs. It cooks up on the stove, almost like an omelet. Feel free to spice things up with ¼–½ teaspoon of your favorite dried herbs or spices.

  ½ cup coconut flour

  6 large eggs

  1 ¼ cup coconut milk

  ½ teaspoon of salt

  1 teaspoon coconut oil

1. In the bowl of a stand mixer, combine the flour, eggs, milk, and salt. Mix on a low speed until smooth.

2. Turn off the mixer and allow the batter to sit for 5 minutes to help the coconut flour absorb the moisture. The batter should be runny. If not, add an extra tablespoon of milk.

3. Place the oil in a skillet with a cover over medium-high heat. Pour ¼ cup of batter onto the skillet and immediately tilt it in different directions to create an 8-inch circle.

4. Place the lid on the skillet and cook for 1–2 minutes, until the edges are golden and slightly turned inward and bubbles form in the middle.

5. Flip the wrap, cover again, and cook another 1–2 minutes or until browned on the other side.

6. Repeat until the batter is used up.

PER SERVING: 55 calories, 5g protein, 3g total fat, 2g total carbohydrate

CHEESY FAUX TORTILLAS

Makes 1 wrap

This is one of the simplest wraps ever! Plus, it is absolutely no carb. While the type of cheese you use for this recipe does not matter, you will need to use deli-style slices. The recipe won't work with chunks you carve off that block of cheddar in your refrigerator.

  2 deli slices of cheese

1. Fold a sheet of parchment paper in half. (You can use a single layer of parchment, but it may be too thin and flimsy to hold the wrap in place when removing from the microwave.)

2. Open the parchment paper and place a single slice of cheese in the center.

3. Slice the second slice of cheese into 8 ribbons.

4. Position the 8 pieces of cheese on the parchment around the large piece of cheese.

5. Lift the parchment with the cheese into a microwave and warm it on medium-high for 12 seconds or until the cheese is barely warm and pliable but not melted.

6. Remove the parchment paper and cheese from the microwave. Using your hand or an oiled rolling pin, fashion the soft cheese into a circle.

7. Place cheese circle in the refrigerator to cool, about 10 minutes.

8. To use, remove the cheese tortilla from the refrigerator and layer it with your favorite fillings, such as homemade Sandwich Salad (page 55). Roll up as you would a regular tortilla.

PER SERVING (USING AMERICAN CHEESE): 160 calories, 8g protein, 14g total fat, 2g total carbohydrate

* If you don't have a microwave, turn your oven to 150–200°F and place the cheese and parchment paper in just until the cheese looks soft. Continue with steps 6–8.

Keto Buns

A lot of people like their sandwiches on rolls or buns—myself included! I am happy to report there are many keto-friendly sandwich buns. Here are my go-to recipes.

EGGPLANT BUNS

Makes 2+ servings

Eggplant is a fun, economical, easy-to-use vegetable for bun-making. This recipe will most likely make more than 2 servings, depending upon how large the eggplant is.

1 eggplant

3 tablespoons ghee, extra-virgin olive oil, avocado oil, or coconut oil, divided

½ teaspoon salt

½ teaspoon pepper

OPTIONAL: ¼ teaspoon of your favorite dried herb or spice

1. Preheat the oven to 425°F. Line a baking sheet with foil and set aside.

2. Slice the eggplant evenly into rounds ¾ inch thick. Arrange in a single layer on the prepared pan.

3. Drizzle half of the ghee evenly over the eggplant, then flip each eggplant slice and drizzle the remaining ghee on the other side. Season with the salt and pepper and optional herbs or spices.

4. Bake the eggplant slices for 18–20 minutes, or until each slice is browned on the outside and just fork-tender. (You don't want to allow these to get mushy or too soft.)

5. Remove from the oven and allow to cool before using. Extras can be stored in a covered container in the refrigerator for up to two days.

PER SERVING: 40 calories, 1g protein, 2g total fat, 1g total carbohydrate

* Chopped-up extra eggplant buns make a great egg sandwich component or addition to scrambled eggs.

PORTOBELLO BUNS

Makes 1 serving

Mushroom buns are very popular in the keto community. If you've never made your own, you're in for a treat: They are easy, come together quickly with few ingredients, and, most important, are outrageously yummy.

½ tablespoon extra-virgin olive oil, avocado oil, or coconut oil

1 clove garlic, minced

1 teaspoon dried oregano

Salt and pepper, to taste

2 portobello mushroom caps, gills removed

1. In a large bowl, whisk together the oil, garlic, oregano, salt, and pepper.

2. Add the mushroom caps to the bowl, and rub the seasoned oil into the caps.

3. Preheat a frying pan to high heat. (You could also use a ridged grill pan.) Add the mushroom caps and cook for 4– 5 minutes on each side, or until fork-tender.

4. Use immediately, or allow to cool before filling with your favorite fillings.

5. Store unused caps in a covered container in the refrigerator for up to 2 days.

PER SERVING: 20 calories, 3g protein, 2g total fat, 2g total carbohydrate

* It is important to clean portobello caps by scraping out the gills. These frills on the underside of the mushroom cap can turn slimy when cooked, and they often hide grit. Using the side of a small spoon, simply scrape them off and discard.

GRILLED ZUCCHINI BUNS

Makes 2 servings

This easy veggie bun recipe uses an indoor grill pan, but you may also choose to use an outdoor grill.

1 tablespoon ghee, extra virgin olive oil, avocado oil, or coconut oil

¼ teaspoon salt

¼ teaspoon pepper

4 (½-inch-thick) slices of a large zucchini

OPTIONAL: ¼ teaspoon of your favorite dried herb or spice

1. In a large bowl, whisk together the ghee, salt, pepper, and optional herbs or spice.

2. Add the zucchini slices and turn to coat.

3. Heat a grill pan over medium-high heat. Lay the zucchini slices on the grill and cook for 2 minutes on each side, or until grill marks are visible and the zucchini is barely fork-tender.

4. Layer with your favorite sandwich fillings.

5. Store unused buns in a covered container in the refrigerator for up to two days.

PER SERVING: 40 calories, 2g protein, 1g total fat, 2g total carbohydrate

SWEET POTATO SLIDER "BUNS"

Makes 4 or 5 servings

Because they have a higher carb content, root veggies aren't eaten often on the keto diet. However, using two slices of sweet potato in place of traditional slider rolls will save you carbs and give you your daily requirement for vitamin A.

1 tablespoon coconut oil, avocado oil, olive oil, or another oil

Salt and pepper, to taste

1-2 large sweet potatoes, sliced ⅓ inch thick

OPTIONAL: Dash of cayenne or chili powder

1. Preheat the oven to 400°F.

2. In a large bowl, whisk together the oil, salt, pepper, and optional spice.

3. Add the sweet potato slices and turn to coat.

4. Arrange the sweet potato slices on a baking sheet.

5. Bake for 12 minutes. Using an offset spatula, turn the slices.

6. Bake for another 12 minutes, or until just fork-tender.

7. Allow to cool before using. Store extra buns in a covered container in the refrigerator for up to two days.

PER SERVING: 80 calories, 2g protein, 1g total fat, 10g total carbohydrate

* When buying sweet potatoes for this recipe, search for ones with a rounder shape and a wider diameter, as they will make better buns.

INSIDE-OUT AVOCADO BURGER POCKETS

This yummy burger features a hidden fatty surprise: avocado! Eat these without a bun or try the Eggplant Buns (page 42).

2 pounds ground beef, bison, or turkey

Salt and pepper, to taste

2 ripe avocados

1 scallion, sliced

½ lemon, juiced

1. In a large mixing bowl, gently combine the ground meat, salt, and pepper. Form eight very thin patties and lay them flat on a tray. Set aside.

2. In another mixing bowl, mash together the avocados, scallion, lemon juice, salt, and pepper.

3. Divide the avocado mixture among four patties, placing a dollop of the mixture in the center of each.

4. Gently position each of the remaining four patties over the avocado-dressed patties to create a burger. Seal the edges of the two patties together, creating four stuffed burgers.

5. Heat a frying pan over medium-high heat. If using turkey, lightly grease the pan with your favorite oil, leftover fat, or butter. Bison and beef have enough fat to prevent sticking to the pan.

6. When the pan is hot, add the four stuffed burgers. Cook about 7–8 minutes or until browned. Gently turn the burger and cook another 7–8 minutes or until done.

7. Remove the burgers from the pan and allow them to rest for 15 minutes. Eat immediately, or wrap with food wrap and refrigerate for up to two days.

PER SERVING: 550 calories, 40g protein, 45g total fat, 5g total carbohydrate

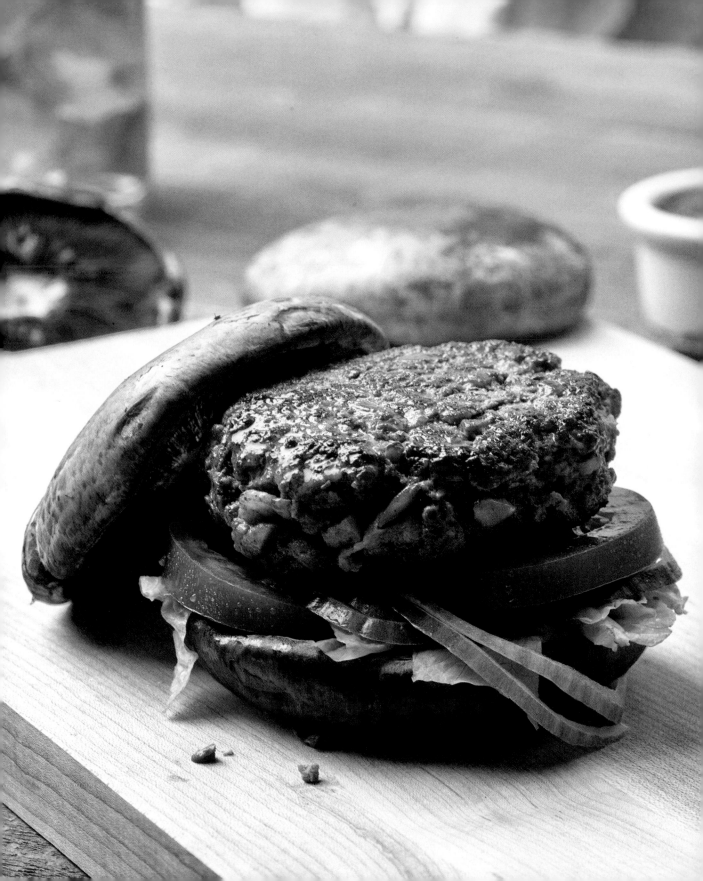

BIG-O BACON BURGERS

Makes 4 servings

Bacon burgers are nothing new, but this one uses bacon in a whole new way: inside the burger, to give it flavor and a moist texture. Serve this burger on a warm Portobello Bun (page 43).

2 tablespoons olive oil, avocado oil, or ghee, divided

½ pound white or cremini (aka baby bella) mushrooms, minced

1 small garlic clove, minced

4 ounces uncooked bacon, roughly chopped

1 pound ground beef, bison, or turkey

1½ teaspoons kosher salt

Freshly ground black pepper

For serving: lettuce, tomato, red onion, and Easy-Peasy Ketchup (page 30)

1. In a large skillet over medium-high heat, warm 1 tablespoon of the oil. Add the mushrooms and garlic and sauté until the liquid they release has cooked off. Set mushrooms aside to cool to room temperature. Wipe down the skillet with a paper towel.

2. Add the bacon to the bowl of a food processor and pulse just until ground.

3. In a large bowl, combine the mushrooms, bacon, and ground bison with salt and pepper. Gently use a spatula or your hands to combine the ingredients.

4. Separate the mixture into four portions and create patties.

5. Return the skillet to the stove over medium heat. Add the remaining oil to the skillet, and when warm, add the four patties. Cook the patties until browned, about 3–4 minutes, and then flip. Cook on the other side about 3–4 minutes or until done.

6. Eat immediately, or place in a covered container in the refrigerator for up to two days.

PER SERVING: 400 calories, 28g protein, 30g total fat, 3g total carbohydrate

KETO SOFT TACOS

A lunchtime favorite from my childhood in Northern California, tacos often wind up in my kids' lunchboxes. Look at the tip for the best way to pack them.

2 egg whites

Pinch of cream of tartar

Dash of cumin or chili powder

½ tablespoon avocado oil, coconut oil, or lard, if cooking poultry

1 pound ground bison, beef, chicken, or turkey

1 garlic clove, minced

1 tablespoon chili powder

1 teaspoon ground cumin

½ teaspoon dried oregano

½ teaspoon salt

OPTIONAL TOPPINGS: Keto Salsa (page 32), Perfect Guacamole (page 25), shredded cheese, and sour cream

1. Make the tortillas: In the bowl of a stand mixer, whisk together the egg whites, cream of tartar, and a dash of cumin or chili powder until the mixture is light. Set aside.

2. Heat a large nonstick skillet over medium heat for 1 minute. Pour in 2 tablespoons of tortilla batter and rotate the pan to help distribute the batter.

3. Cover the pan and cook for 2 minutes. Flip, cover, and cook the tortilla for 2 more minutes.

4. Remove the tortilla and set on a plate. Fold the tortilla in half so it resembles a taco shell and allow to cool.

5. Repeat with the remaining batter. Wipe down the skillet.

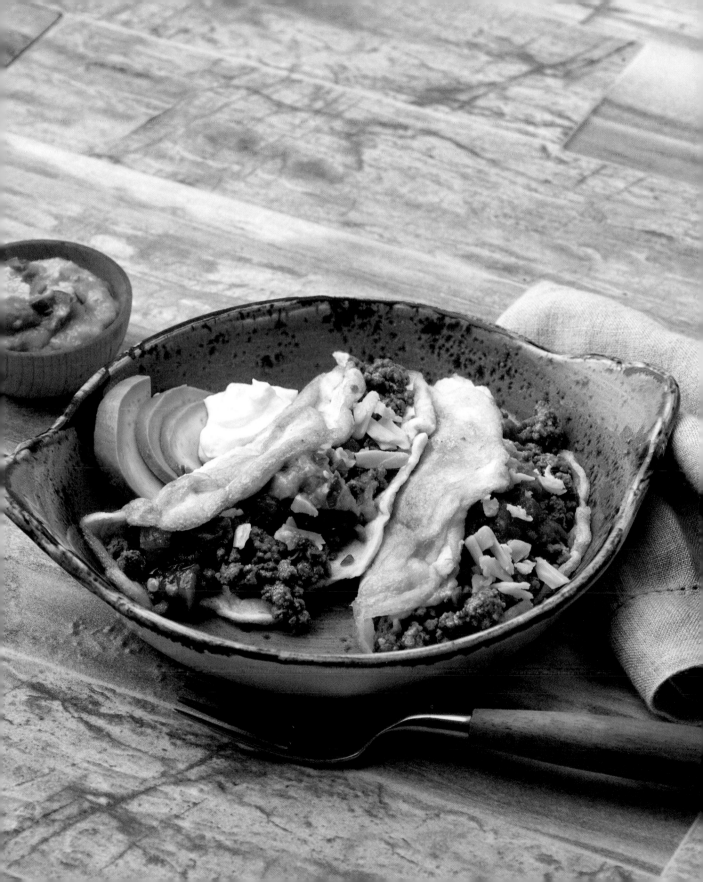

6. Make the taco filling: Return the skillet to medium-high heat. If you will be using ground chicken or turkey, add the avocado oil.

7. Add the ground meat, garlic, chili powder, cumin, oregano, and salt to the skillet and sauté until meat is fully cooked through.

8. Assemble the tacos by holding a tortilla with one hand and filling it with taco meat. Top with optional toppings and eat immediately.

PER SERVING (BEEF TACO, WITHOUT TOPPINGS): 210 calories, 14g protein, 16g total fat, 1g total carbohydrate

＊ If packing these tacos for lunch, wrap the tacos without toppings in foil or food wrap. Store in the refrigerator until ready to eat. Pack the optional toppings in separate small containers.

DELI COUNTER
LETTUCE SUB

The deli sub, a favorite lunchtime option, is a keto no-no when made with a carb-heavy sandwich roll. Use lettuce wraps, however, in place of the bread, and a world of deli-style yumminess is yours. This is a blueprint—feel free to use whatever meats, cheeses, or keto-friendly toppings you have on hand or prefer.

1 large iceberg or butter lettuce leaf
   (see Iceberg Wraps page 38)

1 slice of Muenster or American cheese

3 slices deli ham or roast beef

3 slices deli salami

4 slices deli pepperoni

3 slices deli chicken or turkey

2 pepperoncini peppers, well drained

1 teaspoon Keto Salad Dressing
   (page 22)

1. Lay the lettuce leaf on a flat surface. Layer the cheese, ham, salami, pepperoni, and chicken on the lower third of the lettuce leaf.

2. Top with the pepperoncini peppers, then drizzle the salad dressing over the stack of meat and cheese.

3. Fold in the sides, as if you are making a burrito. Starting at the bottom, roll the leaf as you would a burrito.

4. Wrap in foil or food wrap and store in the refrigerator until ready to eat.

PER SERVING (MADE WITH MUENSTER CHEESE, DELI HAM, AND DELI CHICKEN): 240 calories, 12g protein, 20g total fat, 1g total carbohydrate

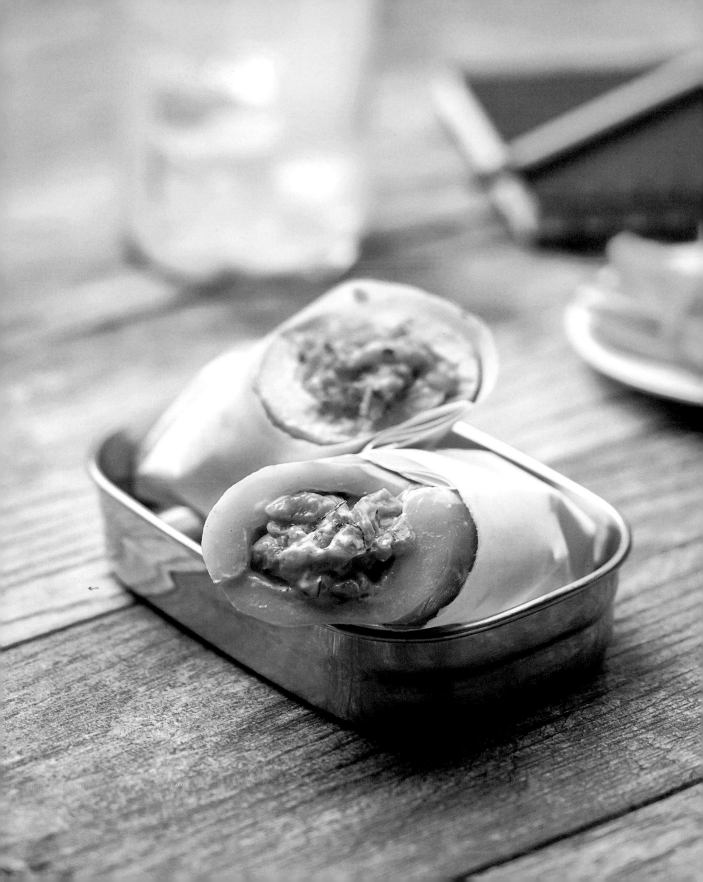

CUCUMBER SUB

Think of this as a ketofied tea sandwich. Feel free to try an equal amount of another protein, such as smoked whitefish, hard-boiled egg (see The Perfect Hard-Boiled Egg on page 8), or leftover chicken.

½ cup chopped smoked trout or smoked salmon

2 tablespoons Housemade Mayo (page 28)

1 teaspoon Dijon mustard

2 teaspoons minced fresh dill

Salt and pepper, to taste

1 cucumber, peeled, halved lengthwise, and seeded

1. In a large bowl, combine all ingredients except the cucumber. Mix gently until combined and adjust seasoning to taste.

2. Fill the center depression in each cucumber half with the fish mixture. Place cucumber halves together, as if they were a hoagie roll. Wrap in food wrap and store in the refrigerator until ready to eat.

PER SERVING (TROUT): 390 calories, 25g protein, 28g total fat, 2g total carbohydrate

＊ To seed a cucumber with ease, run a spoon down the center to scoop out the seedy "marrow."

TRIFLE SANDWICHES

Makes 1 serving

Served in a style similar to the layered dessert, this recipe uses savory sandwich ingredients instead. It's a perfect way to get the taste of a sandwich without wraps or buns or bread.

1 cup Sandwich Salad (facing page), Pulled Pork (page 14), diced Make-Ahead Chicken Thighs (page 11), or diced cooked meat of choice

1 cup shredded romaine lettuce or green cabbage

½ cup Perfect Guacamole (page 25)

½ cup cubed or shredded cheese

OPTIONAL: 1 hard-boiled egg, chopped (see The Perfect Hard-Boiled Egg, page 8)

OPTIONAL: 1 or 2 slices cooked bacon, chopped

1. In a jar, layer ½ cup of the Sandwich Salad or meat, ½ cup of the romaine lettuce, ¼ cup of the guacamole, ¼ cup of the cheese, and all of the optional ingredients.

2. Finish with a second layer of the remaining Sandwich Salad or meat, romaine lettuce, guacamole, and cheese.

CALORIE, FAT, PROTEIN, AND CARBOHYDRATE COUNTS WILL VARY.

SANDWICH SALAD BLUEPRINT

Makes 2 cups, or 4 ½-cup servings

Do you know what Sandwich Salad is? It's not really salad; it's a filling. Think tuna salad, egg salad, chicken salad, or any other kind of chopped-protein-with-fixings kind of sandwich filling. This easy blueprint lets you make a tasty, nutritious, keto-approved sandwich salad no matter what kind of protein you have on hand.

2 tablespoons Homemade Mayo (page 38)

1–3 teaspoons Easy-Peasy Mustard (page 29) or prepared mustard of choice

1–2 tablespoons minced sweet onion (such as Vidalia) or red onion

1–2 tablespoons relish or chopped dill pickles

Salt and pepper, to taste

1½ cups cooked and chopped or flaked protein of choice (such as canned poultry, fish, seafood, red meat, or hard-boiled eggs)

OPTIONAL: 1 or 2 celery stalks, finely chopped

OPTIONAL: 1 or 2 fresh herbs, minced (dill, parsley, cilantro, chives, etc.)

OPTIONAL: Pinch of cayenne, curry, chili powder, or another spice

1. In a large bowl, whisk together all ingredients except the protein.

2. Gently fold in protein of choice, until all ingredients are combined.

3. Serve with a keto-approved wraps or buns or on top of salad greens. Store the remaining Sandwich Salad in a container in the refrigerator for up to two days.

CALORIE, FAT, PROTEIN AND CARBOHYDRATE COUNTS WILL VARY.

＊ If you do not like mayo, consider using 2 tablespoons smashed avocado or Perfect Guacamole (page 25) instead.

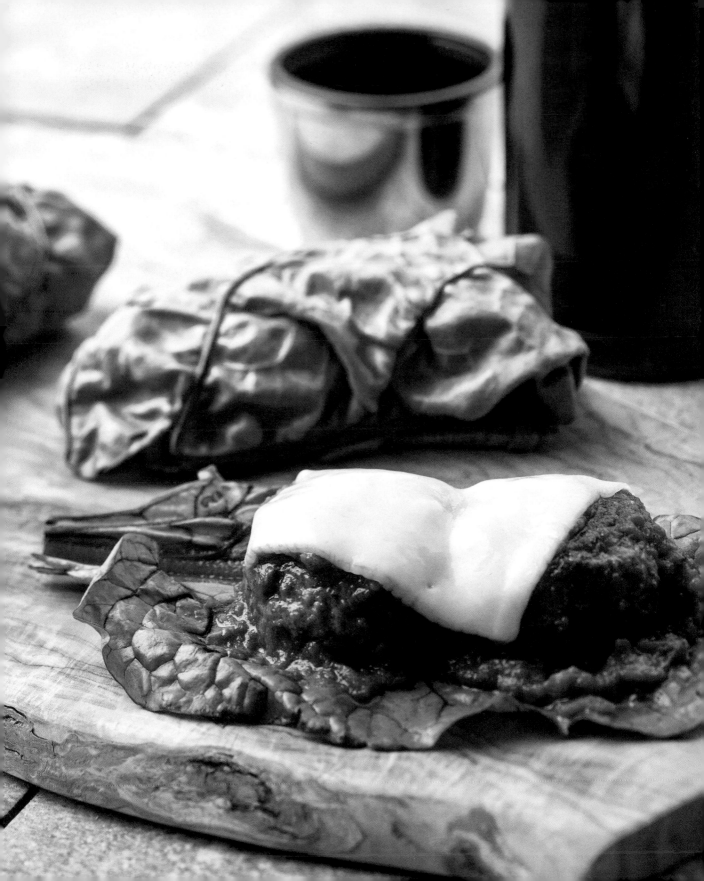

CHARD LEAF MEATBALL HOAGIE WRAP

Chard is related to beet leaves and makes a great sandwich wrapper. You can also use a lettuce wrap if you prefer.

1 large chard leaf

4 Keto Meatballs (page 21)

1 tablespoon Versatile Marinara Sauce (page 26)

1 or 2 slices cheese of your choice

1. Lay the chard leaf on a flat surface. Using a pair of kitchen shears or a knife, remove the stem and about 2 inches of the spine from the leaf. Discard the stem and spine, or chop and sauté as a vegetable for use in another dish.

2. Arrange the meatballs in a horizontal line on the lower third of the leaf, above where you've removed the spine.

3. Top with marinara sauce and cheese.

4. Fold in the two sides, as if you were rolling a burrito.

5. Begin rolling the leaf from the bottom.

6. If necessary, use a toothpick to keep the wrap together. Per serving:

PER SERVING: 590 calories, 20g protein, 22g total fat, 6g total carbohydrate

CHARD LEAF BBQ PULLED PORK HOAGIE WRAP

This wrap works well with Pulled Pork (page 14) as well. Omit the cheese and use a tablespoon of Keto Barbecue Sauce (page 34) in place of the marinara.

* Avoid chard leaves if you have thyroid issues, as they slightly (although temporarily) reduce thyroid function.

PIZZA POCKETS

It is important to use low-moisture cheese when making this pizza-inspired dish. I also suggest using preshredded mozzarella for best results. The instructions seem a bit involved, but these are actually quite easy to make—I promise!

¾ cup shredded mozzarella

1 tablespoon cream cheese

1 tablespoon grated Parmesan

½ teaspoon dried basil

¼ cup flax meal (you can make your own by whirring 1 ounce of flax seeds in a coffee grinder)

8 slices deli salami

4 deli slices provolone

1. Preheat the oven to 400°F.

2. Place a large piece of parchment or wax paper on the counter or another flat surface and have a second, same-size, sheet of parchment or wax paper ready.

3. Place the mozzarella, cream cheese, Parmesan, and basil in a microwave-safe bowl. Microwave on high for about 30 seconds to melt. Check, and if not thoroughly melted, microwave for another 10 seconds, repeating as necessary to melt.

4. Remove from the microwave and stir in the flax meal.

5. Place the dough on the parchment or wax paper. Place the second piece of parchment or wax paper directly on top of the dough.

6. Using a rolling pin, roll the dough out between the two sheets of parchment or wax paper. The dough should be a large rectangle between ⅛ and ¼ inch thick.

7. Cut the rectangle into two squares.

8. Layer the salami and cheese slices on the lower half of each dough square.

9. Fold each square over like an envelope, encasing the ingredients. Press the edges of the dough together to seal.

10. Prick the pockets in a few places to allow the steam to escape while baking.

11. Gently place the parchment with the sealed pizza pockets on an ungreased baking sheet and bake at 400°F for 15–20 minutes, or until golden brown and firm to the touch.

12. Allow to cool on the baking sheet for 15 minutes before cutting in half. Store uneaten pizza pockets in a sealed container in the refrigerator for up to two days.

PER SERVING: 430 calories, 32g protein, 30g total fat, 7g total carbohydrate

CHAPTER THREE

THERMOS LUNCHES

When I was growing up, nothing said homemade lunch like a bottle full of warm goodness. Plus, soup, bisques, chowders, stews, and chilis should be a prominent part of everyone's diet. They are nutritious, comforting, easy to make, and generally economical. These healthy fat-filled warm bowls of broth and hearty ingredients bring back that delicious tradition.

CAULIFLOWER-LEEK BISQUE

Makes 4 servings

Cauliflower soup is one of my absolute favorite soups. Feel free to experiment using your favorite spices or fresh herbs.

2 tablespoons coconut oil

3 tablespoons butter

3 leeks, cleaned and cut into 1-inch pieces

1 large head cauliflower, chopped

3 cloves garlic, finely chopped

8 cups Chicken Bone Broth (page 9)

Salt and freshly ground black pepper, to taste

1 cup heavy cream

1. Add the oil and butter to a large soup pot over medium heat. Add the leeks, cauliflower, and garlic, and sauté for about 10 minutes, or until the vegetables are softened.

2. Stir in the broth and increase the heat to medium-high.

3. Bring the mixture to a boil; then reduce the heat to medium-low, cover, and simmer for 45 minutes.

4. Remove the soup from the heat. Blend the soup with an immersion blender or handheld mixer. Season to taste with salt and pepper. Mix in the cream, and continue blending until smooth.

PER SERVING: 338 calories, 4g protein, 34g total fat, 7g total carbohydrate

MAKE IT VEGAN!

Replace the butter with extra-virgin olive oil or coconut oil, the Chicken Broth with veggie broth, and heavy cream with coconut cream for a plant-based recipe.

BACON-GUACAMOLE SOUP

Makes about 8 servings

This fresh-tasting soup is a bit exotic. Light and refreshing, yet filling and satisfying, it is great for a light meal or enjoyed as a first course. Try it warm, at room temperature, or chilled.

4 cups Chicken Bone Broth (page 9), divided

⅓ cup fresh chopped cilantro, loosely packed

1 large garlic clove, minced

2 medium avocados, peeled and pitted

½ medium lime, juiced

Pinch of cumin

Pinch of chili powder

½ pound bacon, cooked and broken into small pieces

Salt and pepper, to taste

1. Add the broth to a large soup pot over medium-high heat. Bring to a boil, cover the pot, and turn off the heat while prepping the remaining ingredients.

2. Place the cilantro, garlic, avocados, and lime juice in a blender and pulse a few times until chunky.

3. To the blender, add 1 cup of the chicken broth, the cumin, and the chili powder. Blend until smooth.

4. Add the blended mixture to the soup pot with the rest of the broth.

5. Add the bacon to the soup pot.

6. Season with salt and pepper to taste and serve.

7. To serve chilled, allow soup to rest in the refrigerator for a minimum of 90 minutes.

PER SERVING: 290 calories, 15g protein, 22g total fat, 7 g total carbohydrate

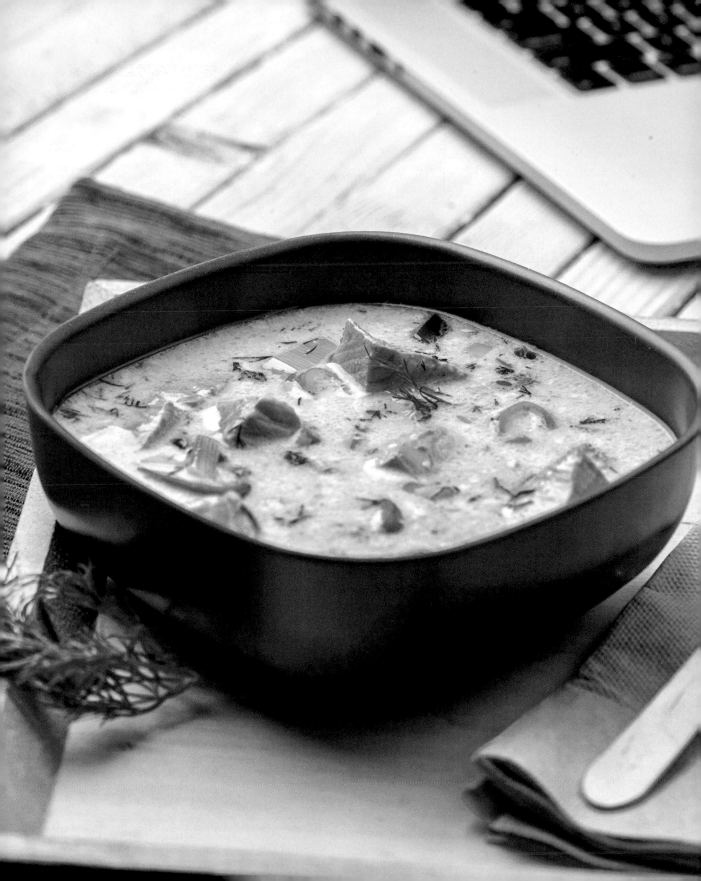

LEEK-AND-SALMON COMFORT CHOWDER

Leeks and salmon together are a winning combination. This creamy chowder is healthy, delicious, comforting, and easy, with only three steps.

2 tablespoons extra-virgin olive oil

4 leeks, washed, trimmed, and sliced into crescents

3 cloves garlic, minced

6 cups Chicken Bone Broth (page 9)

1½ teaspoons dried thyme leaves

1 teaspoon fresh chopped dill (or ½ teaspoon dried)

Salt and pepper, to taste

1 pound salmon fillets or pieces, cut into bite-size pieces (You can use fresh or frozen fish.)

1 (15-ounce) can of coconut milk (about 1¾ cup)

1. Heat the oil in a large saucepan over medium-low heat. Add the leeks and garlic, and cook until slightly softened.

2. Add the broth, thyme, and dill. Simmer for about 15 minutes. Season to taste with salt and pepper.

3. Add the salmon and coconut milk to the pan. Bring back to a gentle simmer and cook just until the fish is opaque and tender. Serve immediately.

PER SERVING: 400 calories, 26g protein, 26g total fat, 7g total carbohydrate

MAKE-IT-YOUR-OWN CHOWDER

Makes 4 servings

This easy fish chowder can be made with fish from last night's dinner, like Fish Baked in Coconut Milk (page 10), or with canned tuna or salmon. You'll come back to this one often!

¼ cup butter or bacon fat

½ cup chopped onion

½ cup chopped celery

½ cup chopped green, red, yellow, or orange bell pepper

1 teaspoon minced garlic

3 cups Chicken Bone Broth (page 9)

1 tablespoon dill, minced (or ½ teaspoon dried)

Salt and pepper, to taste

2 cups heavy cream or coconut cream

3 (6-ounce) cans of tuna or salmon, in oil, or 2 cups of chopped leftover cooked fish of your choice

OPTIONAL: 3 cooked bacon slices chopped and/or ¼ cup of cooked ham, diced

1. Place the butter in a large saucepan over medium heat. When the butter is melted, add the onion, celery, peppers, and garlic, and cook about 5 minutes to soften the vegetables.

2. Add the broth and dill and bring to a boil. Lower the heat, cover, and let simmer for 15–30 minutes.

3. Add the cream and fish—as well as the bacon or ham, if using—and stir to combine. Adjust the salt and pepper to taste. Cook for 5 minutes to combine the flavors.

CALORIE, FAT, PROTEIN, AND CARBOHYDRATE COUNTS WILL VARY.

* Consider using crab, shrimp, or other shellfish as the fish in this dish. Feel free to play with the veggies, as well.

ITALIAN VEGGIE-PROTEIN SOUP

This is one of those "famous" recipes that have been floating around for years and years. The veggies listed below are especially low carb, but this soup can be made with whatever veggies you have on hand. The soup freezes well, making it a great choice for those of you who like to have prepared meals.

2 slices uncooked bacon, chopped

½ tablespoon extra-virgin olive oil

¼ cup chopped onion

1 tablespoon minced fresh garlic

¼ cup chopped sun-dried tomatoes in oil

½ cup sliced white or baby bella mushrooms

4 cups Chicken Bone Broth (page 9)

1 ½ cups water

1 cup peeled and chopped celery root (½ inch cubes)

2 cups chopped cooked chicken breast

1 cup sliced and quartered yellow squash (They will look like small triangles.)

½ cup sliced green beans (1-inch pieces)

2 cups chopped chard (any color)

1 tablespoon red wine vinegar

Salt and pepper, to taste

¼ cup chopped fresh basil

1. In a large soup pot, cook the bacon in the olive oil over medium heat for 2 minutes.

2. Add the onion, garlic, sun-dried tomatoes (with any oil), and mushrooms. Cook for 5 minutes.

3. Pour in the broth and water, then add the celery root and chicken. Simmer for 15 minutes.

4. Add the squash, green beans, and chard and simmer for 10 minutes.

5. Add the red wine vinegar and season with salt and pepper to taste.

6. Stir in the fresh basil just before serving

PER SERVING: 136 calories, 17g protein, 4g total fat, 5g total carbohydrate

ITALIAN WEDDING SOUP

The lovely soup of white beans, escarole, and sausage or meatballs can be easily ketofied. Follow the recipe for Italian Veggie-Protein Soup, replacing one pound of bulk Italian sausage (sweet or hot) for the bacon in step 1. Increase the onion to ½ cup, and omit the sun-dried tomatoes, chopped celery root, chicken breast, yellow squash, green beans, and chopped chard. Instead, add 3 or 4 cups chopped escarole and 1 cup chopped fresh basil leaves in step 4. Enjoy as-is or with as much grated Parmesan cheese as you like.

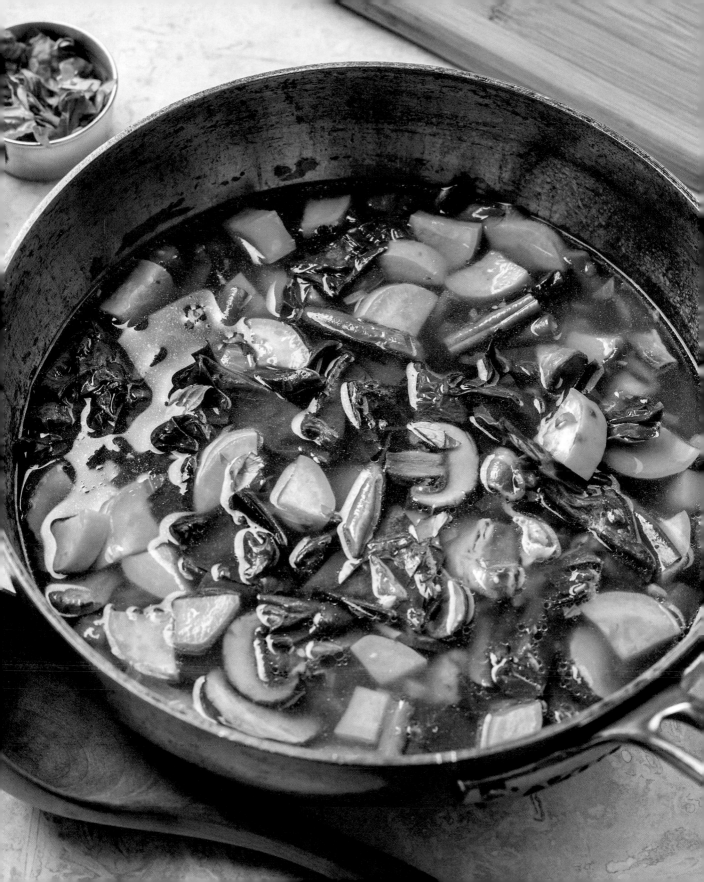

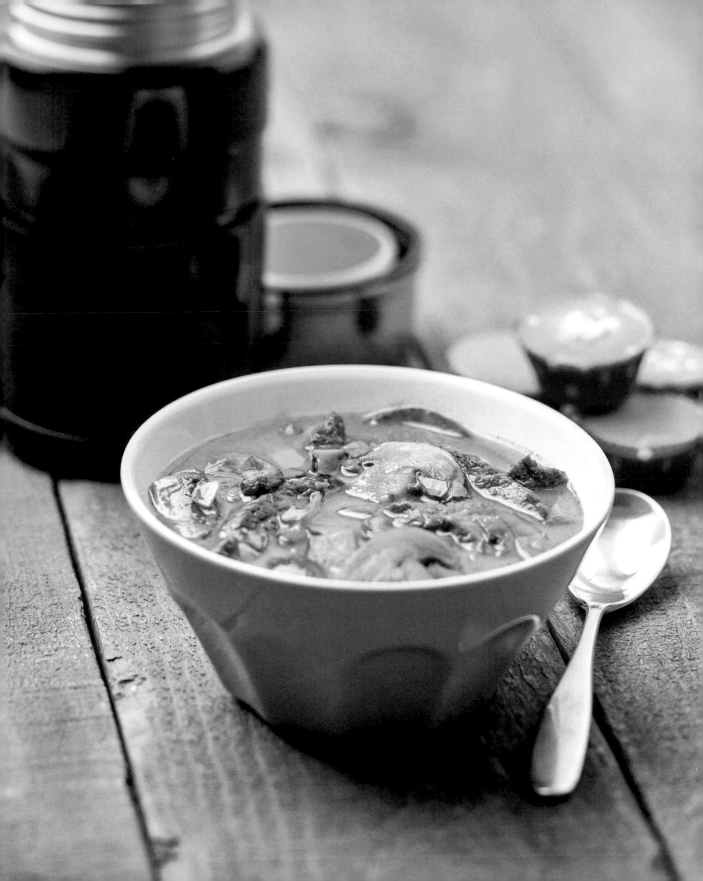

BEEF STROGANOFF STEW

My husband loves Hungarian food, and I spoil him with this delicious stew. When enjoyed for lunch at work, it will make your officemates swoon.

2 large beef rump (sirloin) steaks (about TK pounds)

Salt and pepper, to taste

¼ cup extra-virgin olive oil or ghee, divided

1 medium onion, chopped

2 cloves garlic, minced

1½ pounds white or brown mushrooms, thinly sliced (about 8 cups)

2 teaspoons sweet paprika

1 tablespoon Dijon mustard

5 cups beef bone broth

Juice from 1 large lemon, about ¼ cup

1½ cups whipping cream, coconut cream, or sour cream

¼ cup chopped fresh parsley

1. Slice the steaks into thin, bite-size strips (see tip).

2. Season the steak with salt and pepper to taste.

3. Add half of the olive oil to a large frying pan over medium-high heat. Working in batches, quickly brown the meat on both sides and remove to a waiting plate. Repeat until all the meat has been browned. Set aside.

4. Heat the remaining oil in a heavy soup pot over medium-high heat. Add the chopped onion and minced garlic, and cook until lightly browned and fragrant, about 2–3 minutes.

5. Add the mushrooms and cook for 3–4 more minutes, stirring occasionally.

＊ Pack this soup with Simple Nut Butter Fudge (page 146).

6. Whisk in the paprika, mustard, broth, and lemon juice and bring to a boil. Immediately lower the heat to medium and cook for 2–3 minutes.

7. Add the browned beef slices and whipping cream, and immediately remove the pot from the heat.

8. Stir in the chopped parsley and adjust the seasonings.

PER SERVING: 500 calories, 35 g protein, 39g total fat, 8 g total carbohydrate

* Raw beef is easier to slice thinly when it is partially frozen. Place the beef, unwrapped and in a single layer, in the freezer for 45 minutes before slicing.

KETO CROCKPOT STEW BLUEPRINT

People who often make up fantastic homemade soups with no recipes are sometimes afraid to try their hands at stew-making, but it is quite easy—especially if you let your slow cooker do most of the work. Here's a quick blueprint for a 4- to 6-serving stew to get you started.

2 pounds beef, lamb, pork, or venison stew meat, cut into 1-inch cubes

OPTIONAL: 1–4 slices uncooked bacon, roughly chopped

½ teaspoon salt

½ teaspoon ground black pepper

1–4 cloves garlic, minced

1 teaspoon Worcestershire sauce or soy sauce

1 cup chopped onion, leeks, or shallots

1½ cups Chicken, Bone Broth (page TK), beef broth, or pork broth.

2 cups cauliflower, cut into small florets

2 cups chopped turnip, kohlrabi, rutabaga, or radish (or a combination)

2 stalks celery, chopped

1–2 cups roughly chopped or sliced mushrooms, any kind

1 bay leaf

1 teaspoon paprika

OPTIONAL: ½–1 teaspoon cumin, basil, thyme, oregano

1. Place all ingredients in a slow cooker and stir.

2. Cover, and cook on the low setting for 10–12 hours.

calorie, fat, protein, and carbohydrate counts will vary.

NEW MEXICAN PORK STEW

Makes about 8 servings

This delicious green chile–laced pork stew is a great, filling lunch. Plus, the recipe makes a lot, which is actually a good thing: You'll want to freeze some for later.

3 tablespoons extra-virgin olive oil

2 pounds pork loin, cubed

½ cup chopped onion

2 cloves garlic, minced

1 (2-ounce) can whole Hatch green chiles with liquid

2 teaspoons ground cumin

2 teaspoons granulated garlic

1 teaspoon pure powdered chiles, such as chipotle, ancho, etc.

2 cups low-sodium chicken broth (Regular chicken broth will make the stew too salty.)

Salt and pepper, to taste

OPTIONAL: Chopped cilantro

1. Add the oil to a large sauté pan over medium-high heat.

2. Working in small batches, add the cubed pork loin, browning on all sides but not cooking through. Remove to a waiting platter.

3. Meanwhile, add the onion, minced garlic, and chiles with their liquid to a food processor and pulse into a chunky paste. Set aside.

4. Place a large saucepan on the stove over medium-low heat. Add the browned pork, cumin, granulated garlic, and powdered chiles. Add the pureed chile mixture and broth.

5. Cover the pot with the lid ajar and turn the heat down to low. Cook for 1 ½ hours or until the liquid has cooked down and the pork is tender.

6. Adjust the seasonings, if desired. Garnish with cilantro and serve.

PER SERVING: 185 calories, 19g protein, 11g total fat, 4g total carbohydrate

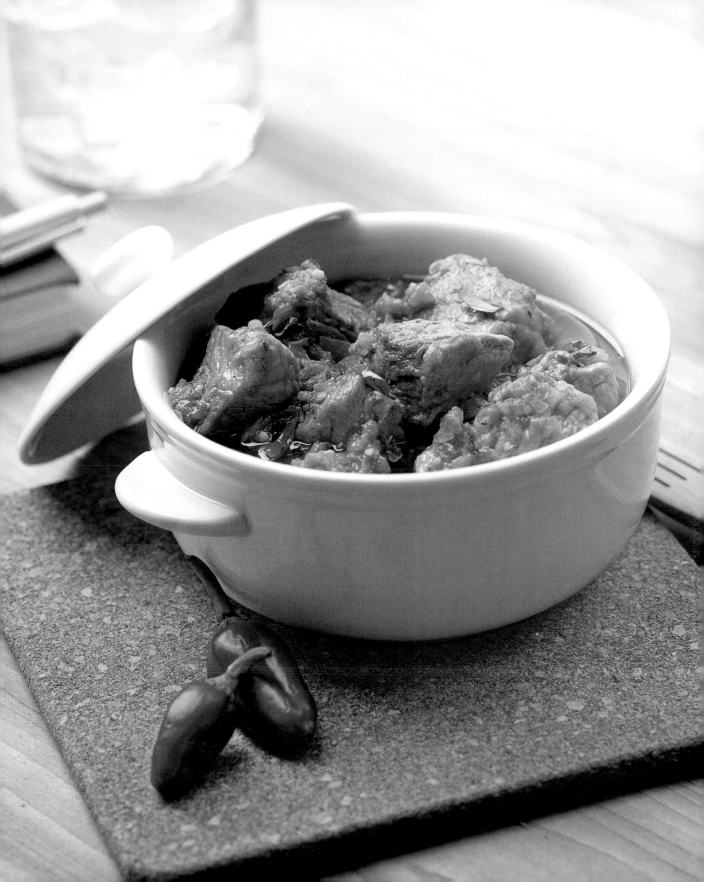

CREAMY SPINACH SOUP

Makes 3 servings

It's easy for keto eaters to forget how important vegetables are to a healthy diet. Spinach is a great low-carb veggie and blends beautifully into soups, like this creamy version.

½ cup butter

½ cup onion, chopped

2 cloves garlic, minced

1 (10-ounce) package frozen, chopped spinach

4 cups Chicken Bone Broth (page 9)

2 teaspoons dried basil

1 teaspoon pepper

1 teaspoon salt

½ cup heavy cream

1. Add the butter to a large soup pot over medium heat.

2. Add the onion and garlic and cook until tender.

3. Stir in the frozen spinach (no need to defrost), chicken broth, basil, pepper, and salt. Increase the heat to medium-high and bring the mixture to a boil.

4. Once the mixture is boiling, decrease the heat to medium-low and allow to simmer for about 10 minutes, or until thickened.

5. Remove the soup from the heat. Blend the soup with an immersion blender or handheld mixer. Mix in the cream and continue blending until smooth.

PER SERVING: 250 calories, 6g protein, 25g total fat, 4g total carbohydrate

MAKE IT VEGAN!

If you'd like to try a vegan, keto-friendly version of this recipe, replace the butter with coconut oil, the Chicken Bone Broth with veggie broth, and the heavy cream with coconut cream.

FATABULOUS KETO CREAM SOUP BLUEPRINT

Makes about 2 to 4 servings

Here's a fast and easy four-serving blueprint. Personalize it however you'd like or ad lib based on what you have on hand.

3 tablespoons fat of choice, such as butter, ghee, avocado oil, coconut oil, lard, bacon grease, olive oil, etc.

1–3 garlic cloves, minced

¼–½ cup chopped leeks, onions, or shallots

¼ cup chopped celery, carrots, and/or bell peppers

2 cups Chicken Bone Broth or beef broth (page TK) or another type of broth

1 cup of heavy cream or coconut cream

Salt and pepper, to taste

¼–1 teaspoon spices, such as cumin, paprika, basil, oregano, etc.

1–3 cups chopped cooked seafood, poultry, or meat

OPTIONAL: 1–3 tablespoons chopped fresh herbs of choice

1. Heat the fat in a large soup pot over medium heat. Add the garlic, leeks, and celery (and/or carrots and/or bell peppers) and cook until soft.

2. Add the broth and allow to simmer for 15–20 minutes.

3. Stir in the cream, salt, pepper, spices, and chopped seafood, poultry, or meat. Adjust the seasonings and cook for 5–10 minutes to blend the flavors.

4. Remove from the heat and stir in the herbs, if using.

CALORIE, FAT, PROTEIN, AND CARBOHYDRATE COUNTS WILL VARY.

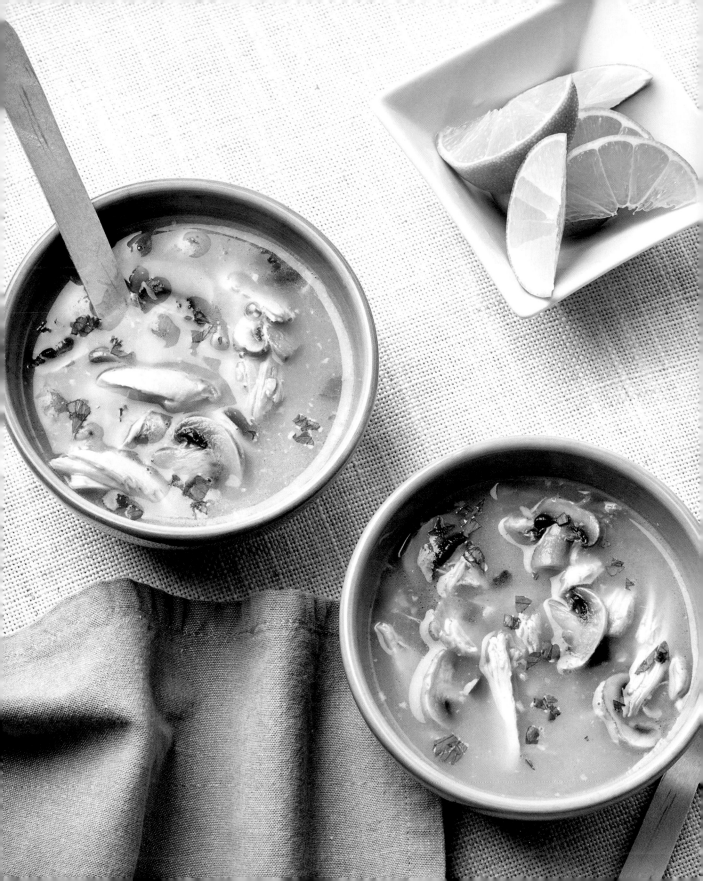

THAI COCONUT SOUP

This recipe for *Tom Kha Gai,* one of Thailand's famous chicken soups, also tastes great with shrimp or pork. You can purchase makrut leaves in the international section of a well-stocked grocery store or online.

6 cups Chicken Bone Broth (page 9)

2 stalks lemongrass

10 makrut lime leaves (or 1 lime)

1 (1-inch) piece fresh ginger, peeled and grated or minced

1 teaspoon soy sauce, or to taste

¾ cup sliced white or mixed mushrooms

½ Serrano or jalapeño chile, chopped

2 cups shredded chicken thigh meat, or chopped cooked shrimp or pork

1½ cups coconut cream

1 tablespoon fish sauce

2 tablespoons chopped cilantro

OPTIONAL: Lime wedges for serving

1. Add the broth to a large soup pot over medium-high heat.

2. Whack the lemongrass stalks with the blunt end of a knife a few times to help release their aroma, then cut the stalks into 1-inch pieces. Add them to the chicken broth along with the makrut lime leaves, ginger, and soy sauce.

3. Simmer the broth for about 20 minutes. Strain out the solids using a strainer, such as a spider, or pour the broth into a colander set over a large bowl and then return the strained broth to the soup pot.

4. Add the mushrooms and chile to the broth and cook for 10 minutes.

5. Add the chicken, coconut cream, and fish sauce and cook for about 5 minutes.

6. Stir in the cilantro and adjust the seasonings if necessary. Divide soup among 4 bowls and serve with lime wedges.

PER SERVING: 350 calories, 19g protein, 21g total fat, 6g total carbohydrate

SIGNATURE TOMATO SOUP

Customized this soup with your favorite spices. Try basil and extra garlic, cumin and curry, or chile powder and fresh cilantro.

2 tablespoons extra-virgin olive oil, butter, coconut oil, or other fat

1 medium onion, chopped

1 stalk celery, chopped

2 cloves garlic, chopped

3 (14-ounce) cans whole peeled tomatoes, with juice

4 cups Chicken Bone Broth (page 9)

½ cup coconut cream

Salt and pepper, to taste

OPTIONAL: 1 teaspoon or more chopped fresh herb of choice, such as thyme, parsley, dill, or cilantro

OPTIONAL: 1 teaspoon or more of your favorite spice, such as cumin, chili powder, or coriander

1. Heat the oil in a Dutch oven over medium heat. Add the onion and celery, and cook, stirring occasionally, until softened, 4–6 minutes. Add the garlic, herbs (if using), and spice (if using), and cook, stirring, until fragrant, about 10 seconds.

2. Stir in the tomatoes. Add the broth, and bring to a lively simmer over high heat. Reduce the heat to maintain a lively simmer and cook for 10 minutes.

3. Stir in the coconut cream, salt, and pepper.

4. Puree the soup in the pot using an immersion blender or in batches if using a blender.

PER SERVING: 195 calories, 5g protein, 14g total fat, 14g total carbohydrate

* Use caution when pureeing hot liquids, always adding to a blender or food processor in small amounts and processing on lower speeds.

CREAM OF TURKEY SOUP WITH BACON

Can you ever have enough cream-based soups? You can use turkey or chicken for this one—I often use it with leftovers from our Thanksgiving bird.

6 slices bacon

2 tablespoons butter

2 cloves garlic, minced

¼ cup sliced mushrooms (button, cremini, shiitake, etc.)

4 ribs celery, chopped

½ cup coconut milk or almond milk

½ cup heavy cream

3 cups Chicken Bone Broth (page 9)

2–4 cups chopped cooked dark meat turkey

Salt and pepper, to taste

2 tablespoons chopped fresh parsley

1. Add the bacon to a large soup pot over medium heat. Cook until crisp.

2. Remove the bacon, keeping as much grease as possible in the pot. Set the bacon aside.

3. Add the butter, garlic, mushrooms, and celery to the pot, and cook until the vegetables are softened.

4. Stir in the coconut milk, heavy cream, and broth.

5. Add the turkey and salt and pepper to taste. Simmer until heated throughout.

6. Chop the bacon and add it, along with the parsley, to the soup.

PER SERVING: 250 calories, 19g protein, 19g total fat, 5g total carbohydrate

CHAPTER FOUR

FATTY BOWLS

I am an enormous fan of bowls. In fact, you'll find at least one bowl recipe in each of my cookbooks. What do I love about them? Well, they are portable, versatile, economical, and even healthy—at least if you use ingredients that support your diet. The recipes in this chapter run the gamut from salad-inspired dishes to heartier fare, all perfect for us keto eaters. Enjoy!

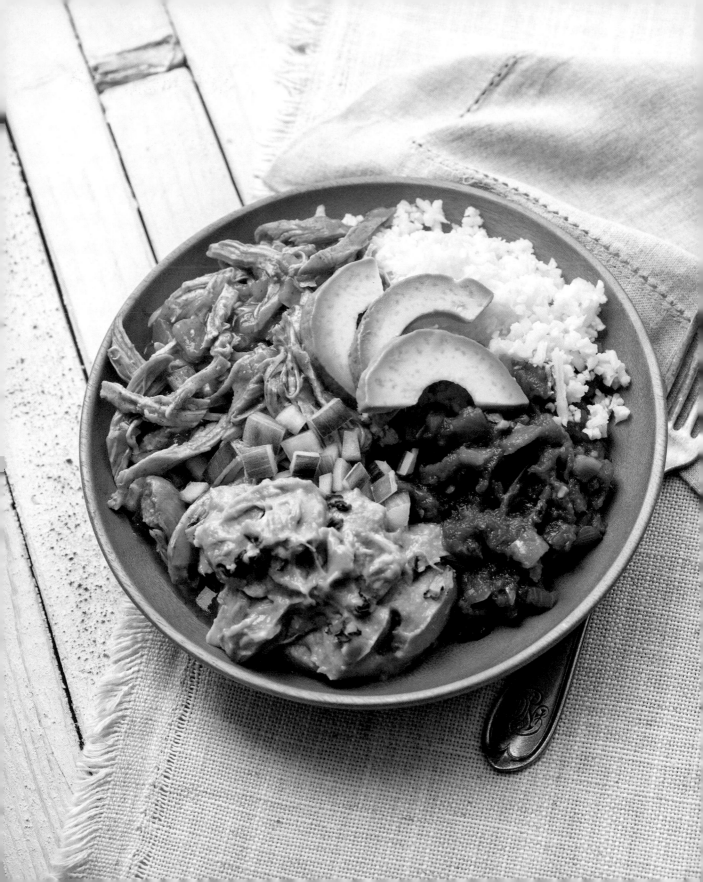

KETO CHICKEN ENCHILADA BOWL

Makes 2 servings

Go ahead and personalize this dish by changing the veggies and seasonings.

2 uncooked chicken breasts

¾ cups prepared red enchilada sauce

1 (4-ounce) can green chiles

¼ cup chopped red onion

¼ cup Chicken Bone Broth (page 9)

1 (12-ounce) bag cauliflower rice (or see recipe on page 111)

Salt and pepper, to taste

Preferred toppings, such as chopped cilantro, sliced avocado, Perfect Guacamole (page 25), shredded cheese, Keto Salsa (page 32), etc.

1. Place a sauté pan over medium heat. In the dry, hot pan, sear all sides of the chicken breasts until lightly browned.

2. Add the enchilada sauce, chiles, onions, and chicken broth to the sauté pan with the chicken. When the mixture begins to simmer, lower the heat to medium-low and cover the pan. Cook until the chicken is tender, about 10 minutes. Turn off the heat and remove just the chicken.

3. Place the chicken in a large bowl. Shred the chicken using two forks. Add the shredded chicken back to the sauce in the sauté pan and turn the heat to medium. Allow the mixture to simmer for 10 minutes or until any liquid has disappeared. Remove from the heat and set aside.

4. Meanwhile, prepare the cauliflower rice per the bag's instructions and dice your preferred toppings.

5. To assemble the bowls: Place the cauliflower rice in the bottom of a sealable food container. Layer with the chicken mixture. Top with toppings of your choice. Seal and place in the refrigerator for up to three days.

PER SERVING: 200 calories, 19g protein, 10g total fat, 5g total carbohydrate

KETO POKE-ISH BOWL

Makes 2 servings

This keto-friendly version of the trendy Hawaiian dish does not use raw fish, which may not store well in your office refrigerator. Instead, it uses cooked salmon or tuna—or any leftover seafood or protein you may have in your refrigerator.

1 tablespoon rice wine vinegar

2 tablespoon sesame oil

1 teaspoon fish sauce

Salt and pepper, to taste

2 cups cooked Broccoli Rice

1 English cucumber, peeled and chopped

1 celery stalk, chopped

1 cup sliced snow peas

2 radishes, sliced

1 carrot, peeled and shredded

1 cup watercress or other greens

2 cups cooked salmon, such as leftover Fish Baked in Coconut Milk (page 19), cut or flaked into bite-size pieces

OPTIONAL: 2 tablespoons chopped cilantro, parsley, or dill

1. In a small bowl, whisk together the vinegar, oil, fish sauce, salt, and pepper. Set the dressing aside.

2. To assemble the bowls: Divide the broccoli rice between two sealable containers. Layer the cucumber, celery, snow peas, radishes, carrot, and watercress, dividing between the two containers.

3. Drizzle the dressing over the contents of both containers.

4. Divide the fish between the two containers, placing it directly on top of the dressed vegetables.

5. Sprinkle the herbs, if using, over the top of each container before sealing each with a lid. Place in the refrigerator for up to two days.

PER SERVING (WITHOUT OPTIONAL INGREDIENTS): 500 calories, 30g protein, 40g total fat, 15g total carbohydrate

WHAT ELSE CAN YOU USE?
You can use cooked tuna or another fish in place of salmon. Canned fish works, as well.

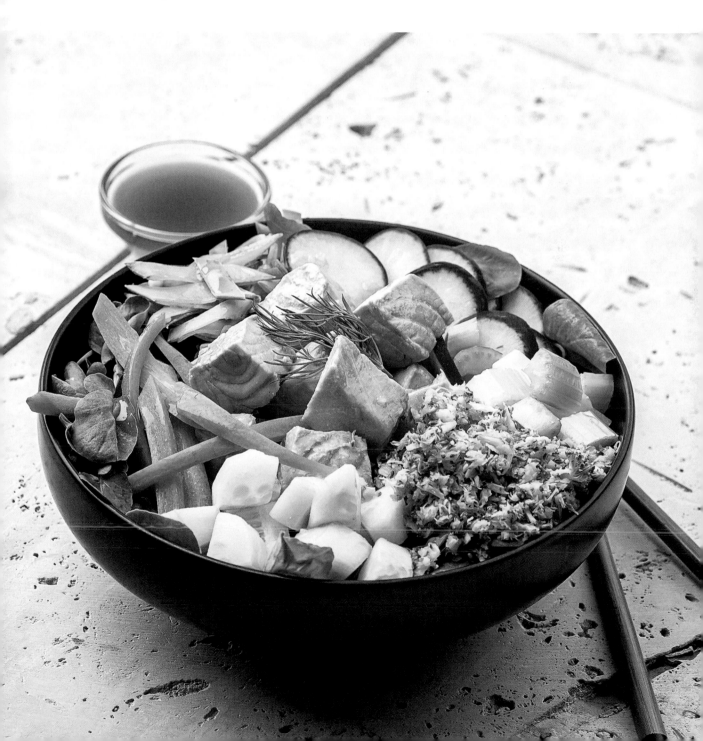

KETO BOWL BLUEPRINT

As a keto eater, you know that those trendy grain and bean bowls are way too carb-heavy to fit into your eating plan. Fortunately, there is an easy way to enjoy a lunch bowl in a keto-approved way: make your own!

 You can put together a bowl with just about anything you have in your kitchen—even if you only have small amounts of this and that. Plus, bowls are super portable—just layer the ingredients in a Mason jar or a grab-and-go container and toss it into your bag, and you've got an easy lunch. Follow this blueprint.

Makes 1 serving

¼ cup (or more) Keto Salad Dressing (page 22), or your favorite salad dressing

1 tablespoon (or more) favorite herb or mix of herbs

1 garlic clove, minced

¼ cup minced red onion, scallions, or shallots

Salt and pepper, to taste

1 avocado, chopped

2 cups cooked (or canned) fish, seafood, poultry, or red meat of your choice

2 cups chopped cooked or raw vegetables, such as Cauliflower Rice (page 111) or broccoli stems

OPTIONAL: ½ cup shredded or cubed cheese

OPTIONAL: 1 hard-boiled egg, chopped (see The Perfect Hard-Boiled Egg, page 8)

OPTIONAL: 1–2 slices of bacon, cooked and chopped

OPTIONAL: ½ cup or more shredded unsweetened coconut

1. In a lunch container or jar, add the salad dressing, herbs, garlic, onion, salt, and pepper and whisk or shake until the ingredients are combined.

2. Add the avocado to the dressing and toss gently until coated. Adjust the salt and pepper to taste.

3. Add all the other ingredients on top of the dressing. Do not stir! Allow the dressing and avocado to sit at the bottom of the container until you're ready to eat.

4. Place the lid on the container and store in the refrigerator.

5. Before eating, shake the container gently to distribute the dressing.

CALORIE, FAT, PROTEIN AND CARBOHYDRATE COUNTS WILL VARY.

KETO GREEK SALAD

Makes 2 servings

Greek salad is a universal favorite—plus it is keto-friendly! If you'd like more protein, feel free to add a cup of grilled chicken, lamb, or squid.

½ large, seedless English cucumber (about 6–7 ounces), chopped

½ red bell pepper, chopped

1 cup halved cherry or grape tomatoes

⅓ cup Kalamata olives

¼ small red onion, thinly sliced

3 ounces feta, cubed

2 tablespoons extra-virgin olive oil, or more to taste

1 tablespoon red wine vinegar

1 teaspoon fresh oregano (or ½ teaspoon dried)

Salt and freshly ground black pepper to taste

1. In a large bowl, combine the cucumber, pepper, tomatoes, olives, onion, and feta.

2. In a small bowl, whisk together the olive oil, vinegar, oregano, salt, and pepper to make a dressing.

3. Pour the dressing over the salad right before serving. If packing the salad, store the salad and dressing separately.

PER SERVING: 380 calories, 45g protein, 33g total fat, 17g total carbohydrate

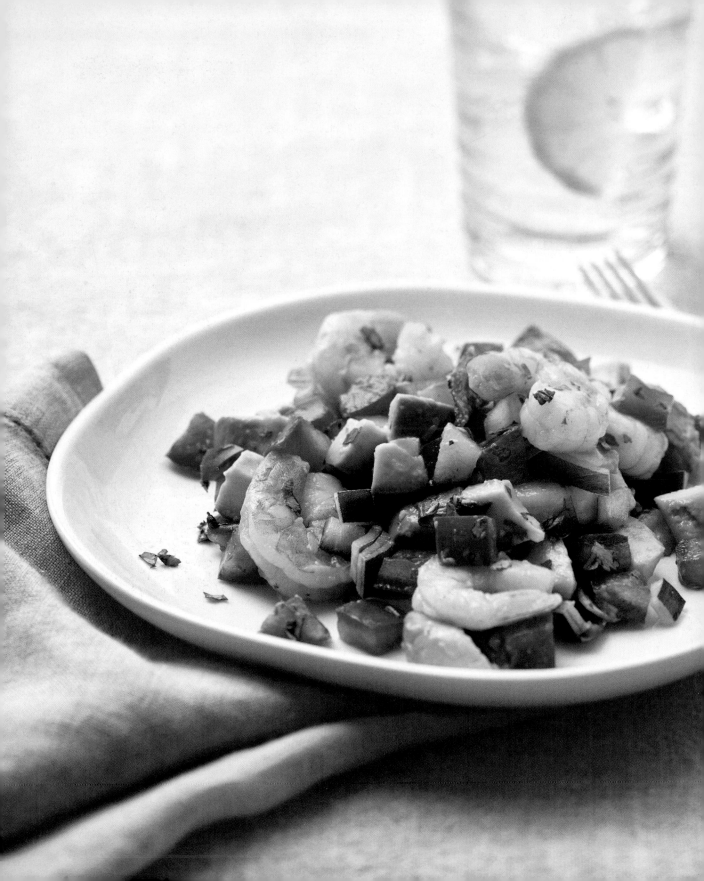

AVOCADO-SHRIMP SALAD

Makes 2 servings

Shrimp and avocado are a beautiful pairing of protein and fat and great for keto eaters. This luxurious lunch salad travels well and can be customized with the addition of extra veggies.

¼ cup chopped red onion

2 limes, juiced

1 tablespoon avocado or extra-virgin olive oil

Pinch of salt

Pinch of pepper

1 pound cooked large or jumbo shrimp, peeled, deveined, and tails removed

1 avocado, diced

1 medium tomato, cored, seeded, and diced

1 jalapeño, seeds removed, minced

1 tablespoon chopped cilantro

1. In a small bowl, combine the onion, lime juice, oil, salt, and pepper. Let the onion marinate for at least 5 minutes to mellow its flavor.

2. In a large bowl, combine the shrimp, avocado, tomato, and jalapeño.

3. Add the onion–lime juice mixture to the shrimp mixture. Add the cilantro and gently toss. Adjust the salt and pepper to taste.

PER SERVING: 380 calories, 45g protein, 17g total fat, 14g total carbohydrate

* You can use the shrimp whole, but I like to chop them so I get a piece of shrimp in each bite.

CAULIFLOWER-TABBOULEH SALAD

Makes 6 servings

Traditional tabbouleh uses bulgur, a wheat product that's filled with gluten, which can set off eczema—not to mention all the carbs. This fun, yummy version uses riced cauliflower. Feel free to add chopped poultry or salmon.

Florets from 1 large head cauliflower

½ cup lemon juice

¾ cup extra-virgin olive oil

1 bunch parsley or cilantro, washed and chopped

1 bunch green onions (also known as scallions), chopped

2 cups chopped Roma tomatoes

1 teaspoon salt

1 teaspoon pepper

1. Add the cauliflower florets to a food processor and pulse until they resemble rice.

2. In a large bowl, combine the cauliflower and lemon juice and stir well.

3. Add the olive oil, parsley, green onions, tomatoes, salt, and pepper.

4. Stir well.

5. Taste and add more salt and pepper if needed.

6. Cover and refrigerate for at least 4 hours, stirring once each hour.

PER SERVING: 155 calories, 4g protein, 9g total fat, 15g total carbohydrate

* Look for prepared cauliflower rice at your supermarket in the produce section for a time saver.

BARBECUE SALAD

Makes 2 servings

This fun salad is for all of you pulled-chicken and pulled-pork sandwich aficionados. Feel free to fatify this further by adding a diced avocado or ½ cup of cheese.

¼ cup Keto Barbecue Sauce (page 34)

1 tablespoon mayonnaise

Salt and pepper, to taste

2 cups Pulled Pork (page 14) or Make-Ahead Chicken Thighs (page 11), chopped

2 cups shredded green or savoy cabbage

2 carrots, grated

¼ cup diced red onion

OPTIONAL: hot sauce, to taste

1. In a small bowl, whisk together the barbecue sauce, mayo, salt, pepper, and hot sauce, if using, until emulsified.

2. If you are packing the salad, divide the salad dressing between two lunch containers, pouring half the dressing into the bottom of each container.

3. Next, layer the pork in each container.

4. Place the cabbage, carrots, and onion in a large bowl and toss gently to combine.

5. Place the tossed salad on top of the dressing and pork in each lunch container.

6. Seal immediately and store in the refrigerator.

7. Before eating, shake the container gently to distribute the dressing.

PER SERVING: 400 calories, 30g protein, 33g total fat, 7 g total carbohydrate

KETO COBB SALAD

The dish was created in the 1930s when a hungry restaurant owner named Robert Howard Cobb wanted something to eat. The only ingredients available at his Hollywood restaurant, the Brown Derby, were assembled into a quick salad. It was so delicious, he gave it a name and placed on the menu.

2 tablespoons extra-virgin olive oil or avocado oil

1 tablespoon apple cider vinegar

Salt and pepper, to taste

1 medium avocado, diced

3 slices cooked bacon, minced

1 cup cubed cooked chicken breast

½ cup cubed cheddar cheese

1 large hard-boiled egg, roughly chopped (see The Perfect Hard-Boiled Egg, page 8)

1 head romaine lettuce, roughly chopped

1. Whisk together the oil, vinegar, salt, and pepper until emulsified. Set aside.

2. If packing the salad, divide the salad dressing between two lunch containers, pouring half the dressing into the bottom of each container.

3. Add the diced avocado to the salad dressing in each container.

4. Place all remaining salad ingredients in a large bowl and toss gently to combine.

5. Place the tossed salad on top of the dressing and avocado in each lunch container.

6. Seal immediately and store in the refrigerator.

7. Before eating, shake the container gently to distribute dressing.

PER SERVING: 675 calories, 50g protein, 49g total fat, 8g total carbohydrate

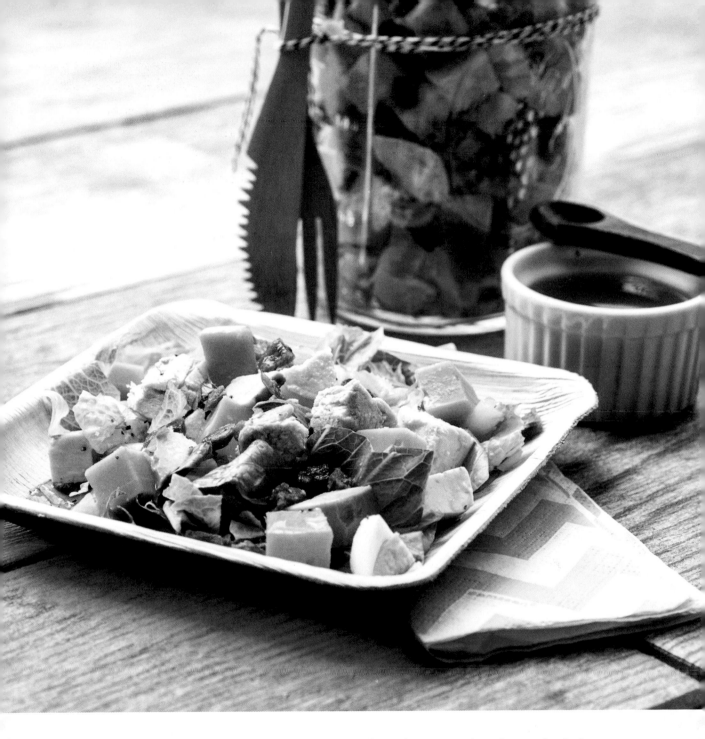

* See the Keto Bowl Blueprint (page 88) to learn how to make a layered salad like the one pictured here.

CHEESEBURGER SALAD

Makes 2 servings

This salad is unusual in that it contains ground beef—something not normally seen on a salad. But as we keto eaters know, ground beef belongs anywhere you want it to. Feel free to use ground bison, pork, sausage, lamb, or venison in place of the beef.

½ pound ground beef

1 garlic clove, minced

Salt and pepper, to taste

¼ cup mayonnaise

1 tablespoon white wine vinegar

1 teaspoon brown or yellow mustard

1 head romaine lettuce, roughly chopped

2 plum tomatoes, roughly chopped

2 scallions, chopped, or ¼ cup diced red onion

½ cup shredded cheddar cheese

¼ cup chopped dill pickles, or chopped pickled jalapeños

1. In a large sauté pan over medium-high heat, cook the ground beef and garlic, seasoning with salt and pepper to taste. Cook until the beef is browned and cooked through, about 8–10 minutes.

2. Using a slotted spoon, remove the beef mixture from the sauté pan and place on a plate or in a bowl. Set aside. Reserve the fat from the pan to use in the dressing.

3. Place the leftover beef drippings, mayonnaise, vinegar, and mustard in a blender or food processor. Pulse until smooth. Add salt and pepper to taste.

4. If taking the salad to work, divide the salad dressing between two lunch containers, pouring half the dressing into the bottom of each container.

5. Place the lettuce, tomatoes, scallions, cheese, and pickles in a large bowl and toss gently to combine.

6. Place the tossed salad on top of the dressing. Add half of the reserved beef mixture on top of the salad ingredients in each container.

7. Seal immediately and store in the refrigerator.

8. Before eating, shake the container gently to distribute the dressing.

* If you've ever wondered, yes, the different grades of ground beef contain different amounts of fat. Sirloin, typically the most expensive, is also the leanest, weighing in at 5–10 percent total fat. The next lean is round, with 10–15 percent total fat. The fattiest (and usually least expensive) is the keto favorite known as ground chuck. It contains 15–20 percent fat. When buying beef, I often opt for the least expensive. If you're a hard-core keto eater, you'll purchase chuck.

PER SERVING: 400 calories, 30g protein, 33g total fat, 7g total carbohydrate

ITALIAN SAUSAGE BOWL

This salad is based on the popular Italian sausage, onion, and pepper sandwich. This yummy salad offers up that delicious, familiar taste we love in a low-carb, keto-friendly bowl.

1 small sweet onion, such as Walla Walla or Vidalia, roughly chopped

1 red, green-or orange bell pepper, roughly chopped

3 tablespoons extra-virgin olive oil, divided

Salt and pepper, to taste

½ pound Italian sausage links, sweet or hot, sliced into coins

1 garlic clove, minced

2 tablespoons red wine vinegar

1 head romaine lettuce, roughly chopped

OPTIONAL: ¼ teaspoon dried basil

OPTIONAL: ¼ teaspoon dried oregano

1. Preheat the oven to 375°F and set out a large rimmed baking pan.

2. In a large bowl, toss the onion, pepper, and herbs, if using, with 1 tablespoon of the olive oil and salt and pepper to taste. Transfer the mixture to the baking pan. Add the sausage pieces.

3. Bake for 15 minutes or until the sausage is browned and the vegetables are soft and beginning to caramelize. Remove from the oven, pour off the drippings (reserve them to be used for the dressing), and set aside the vegetables and sausage.

4. Add the garlic, salt and pepper to taste, the remaining 2 tablespoons of olive oil, red wine vinegar, and the drippings from the baking pan to a blender and process until smooth.

5. If packing the salad, divide the salad dressing between two lunch containers, pouring half the dressing into the bottom of each container.

6. Place the roasted sausage and vegetables in the containers, on top of the salad dressing.

7. Add the lettuce, dividing between the two containers.

8. Seal immediately and store in the refrigerator.

9. Before eating, shake the container gently to distribute the dressing.

PER SERVING: 405 calories, 29g protein, 30g total fat, 10 g total carbohydrate

CHAPTER FIVE

KETO COMFORT FOODS

If you're like many keto eaters, one of the things you miss most is traditional comfort food—saucy, creamy, carby foods that allow us to sink into a blissed-out cocoon. When you are eating keto, however, a plate of spaghetti with your favorite sauce is not a good lunchtime option. Ditto your favorite casserole. Neither is anything with white rice or mashed potatoes or polenta or grits or, or, or . . . Fortunately, this chapter can help you keto-eating comfort food lovers with a range of saucy, yummy, and soothing recipes that are perfect for lunch.

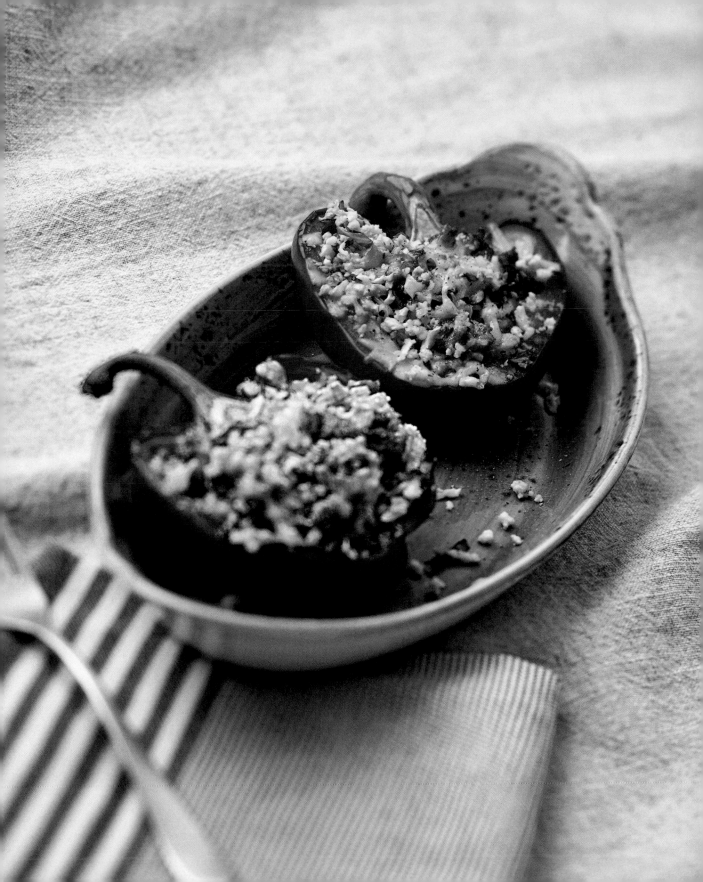

KETO ITALIANO STUFFED PEPPERS

Makes 2 servings

When I was growing up, my mom would occasionally make stuffed peppers using green bell peppers, leftover meatloaf, and instant rice. I like them . . . but I love these even more. Feel free to use a different color pepper if you'd like.

1½ cups small cauliflower florets, raw

1 tablespoon olive oil

1 teaspoon dried basil, or a combination of dried basil and oregano, divided

Salt and pepper, to taste

6 ounces Italian sweet or hot sausage, casing removed

2 large red bell peppers

½ cup grated provolone cheese, divided

1. Preheat the oven to 350°F.

2. Place the cauliflower in a food processor and pulse until it resembles rice. Or use a box grater and grate the cauliflower.

3. Combine the cauliflower rice, olive oil, ½ teaspoon of the basil, salt, and pepper in a sauté pan with a lid and let it steam over medium heat until the cauliflower is tender, for about 6 minutes. Remove the pan from the heat and set aside.

4. In another sauté pan, cook the sausage, the remaining basil, salt and pepper to taste until the sausage is no longer pink. Set aside.

5. Remove the sausage from the pan with a slotted spoon and let drain on paper towels. Reserve the grease.

6. Add the sausage, sausage grease, and cauliflower rice to a large bowl with ¼ cup of the cheese. Stir to combine. Adjust seasonings if necessary. Set aside.

7. Prepare the peppers by carefully cutting off the tops. Then place the peppers on their sides and cut them in half lengthwise. Remove the seeds. You will have four pepper halves.

8. Place the peppers cut side up in a lightly greased baking dish and spoon the sausage-cauliflower mixture into each pepper half. Top with the remaining cheese.

9. Cover the dish with foil and bake for 25 minutes.

10. Remove the foil and bake for 10 more minutes or until the cheese is bubbly.

PER SERVING: 350 calories, 19g protein, 25g total fat, 12 g total carbohydrate

* For a stand-alone recipe for Cauliflower Rice, see page 111.

MEATY FRIED "RICE"

Substitute any type of poultry, red meat, or seafood you have on hand for the pork, if desired.

1 large head cauliflower, separated into florets

2 tablespoons avocado or coconut oil, divided

2 cloves garlic minced

½ medium onion, chopped

1 pound pork chops or pork loin, minced

1 celery stalk, chopped

1 large egg, beaten

2 tablespoons soy sauce

1 teaspoon toasted sesame oil

OPTIONAL: ½ cup frozen peas

OPTIONAL: ½ cup diced red bell pepper

OPTIONAL: ½ cup finely shredded cabbage

1. In the bowl of a food processor, process the cauliflower until it resembles rice. Or, use a box grater and grate the cauliflower. Set aside.

2. Add the oil to a large skillet over medium-high heat. Add the garlic and onion and cook until softened, about 4–5 minutes. Add the pork and cook until barely opaque. Do not overcook at this early stage, as pork will continue to cook as you add the remaining ingredients.

3. Add the riced cauliflower and sauté for 2–3 minutes. Add the celery and any optional vegetables and cook for 1–2 minutes, being careful not to overcook. (You don't want mushy fried rice!)

4. Add the egg, soy sauce, and sesame oil and cook until the egg is scrambled, for about one minute.

5. Enjoy immediately, or pack in a covered container and store in the refrigerator for up to two days.

PER SERVING (WITHOUT OPTIONAL INGREDIENTS): 350 calories, 30g protein, 20g total fat, 12g total carbohydrate

CILANTRO-LIME SHRIMP SCAMPI WITH ZUCCHINI NOODLES

Makes 4 servings

This is a traditional special-occasion recipe that is actually perfect for your workday lunch. Serve over Cauliflower Rice (page 111) or spiralized zucchini noodles.

2 tablespoons coconut oil, extra-virgin olive oil, or butter

1 pound jumbo shrimp (16–24), shelled and deveined

4 cloves garlic, chopped

OPTIONAL: Pinch-red pepper flakes

¼ cup Chicken Bone Broth (page 9)

1 lime, juiced (about 2 tablespoons)

Salt and pepper, to taste

2 tablespoons chopped cilantro

Base of choice, such as spiralized zucchini noodles or Cauliflower Rice

1. Warm the oil in a large sauté pan over medium-high heat. Add the shrimp, cook for 2 minutes, then flip. Add the garlic and red pepper flakes, if using, and cook for 1 more minute before setting the shrimp aside.

2. Add the broth, lime, salt, and pepper to the pan, scrape any browned bits from the bottom of the pan, and simmer for 2 minutes.

3. Return the shrimp to the pan with the cilantro, and toss to combine. Remove from the heat and pour over your base of choice.

PER SERVING (WITH ZUCCHINI NOODLES): 350 calories, 30g protein, 20g total fat, 10g total carbohydrate

∗ Don't own a spiralizer? You can purchase spiralized noodles in the produce section of most grocery stores.

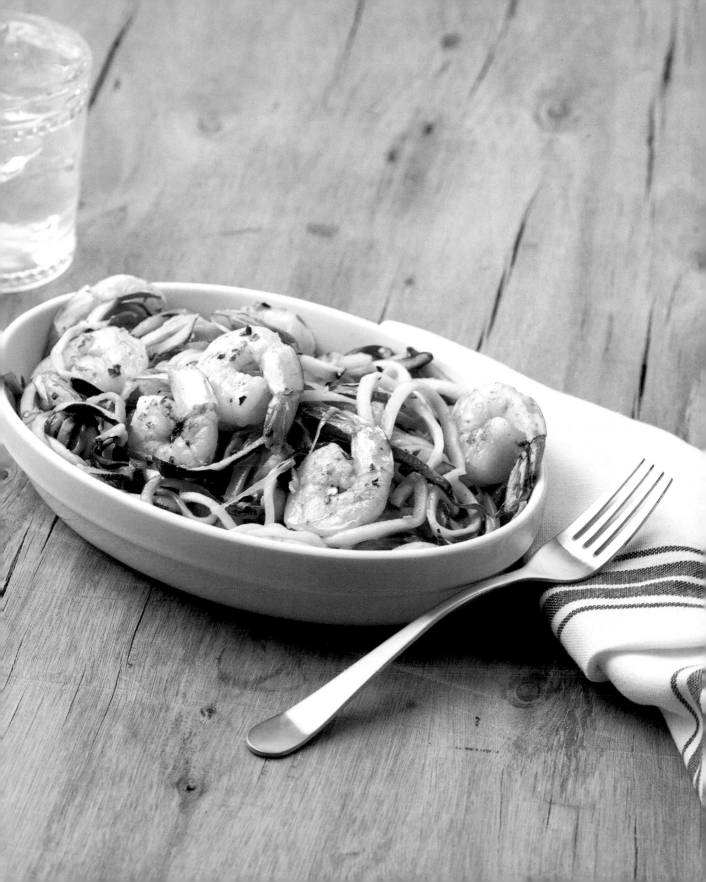

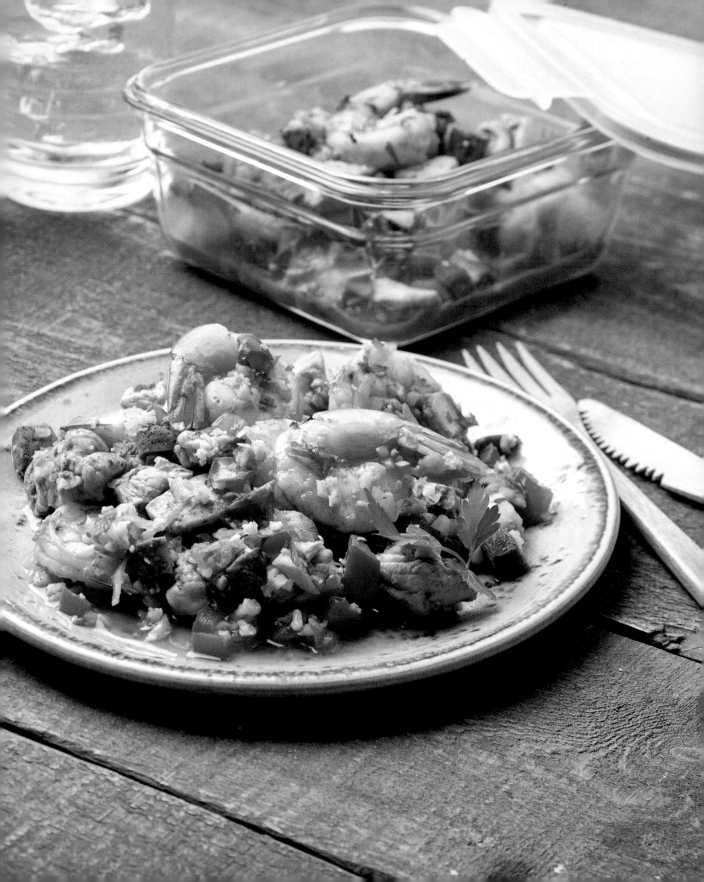

MIXED KETO PAELLA

This take on traditional paella features all the things my family loves about paella, with none of the carb-heavy rice. This recipe can be adjusted based on the proteins and vegetables you have on hand.

1 head cauliflower, separated into florets

¾ cup Chicken Bone Broth (page 9)

2 tablespoons extra-virgin olive oil, divided

4 boneless, skinless chicken thighs, cubed

1 medium yellow onion, chopped

2 cloves garlic, minced

½ red bell pepper, diced

2 Roma tomatoes, chopped

Salt and pepper, to taste

1 teaspoon saffron threads

¼ teaspoon smoked paprika

8 ounces chorizo sausage

½ pound jumbo shrimp, peeled and deveined

¼ cup fresh parsley

Lemon wedges for garnish

1. In the bowl of a food processor, process the cauliflower until it resembles rice. Or, use a box grater and grate the cauliflower. Set aside.

2. Add the broth to a large saucepan over medium heat.

3. Heat 1 tablespoon of the olive oil in a large skillet over medium-high heat. Add the chicken pieces and cook for 5 minutes, stirring occasionally to brown the chicken on all sides.

4. Add the remaining 1 tablespoon of oil, onion, garlic, red pepper, tomatoes, salt, pepper, saffron, paprika, and chorizo. Continue to sauté for another 7 minutes, until the onions have softened.

5. Pour the warm broth into the skillet, stirring to scrape up the browned bits from the bottom of the skillet.

6. Stir in the shrimp and the riced cauliflower and simmer for 5 minutes, or until the shrimp looks done.

7. Sprinkle the parsley over the top. Garnish with lemon wedges.

8. Enjoy immediately or store in a sealed container in the refrigerator for up to two days.

PER SERVING: 490 calories, 40g protein, 30g total fat, 14g total carbohydrate

Faux Rice, Pasta, and Potatoes

If you're like me, one of your favorite parts of a saucy, comfort food meal is the rice, pasta, or potatoes served alongside. When you're on the keto diet, however, these are no-nos. Here are some popular keto-approved side dish substitutions.

CAULIFLOWER RICE

Makes 4 servings

This recipe can be personalized with additional herbs or spices. Have fun with it!

1 large head cauliflower, separated into 1-inch florets

3 tablespoons butter

2 garlic cloves, minced

Salt and pepper, to taste

OPTIONAL: 1–2 teaspoons lemon juice, to keep the cauliflower white

OPTIONAL: 2 tablespoons fresh herbs, such as parsley or chives

1. Add the cauliflower to the bowl of a food processor and pulse until the cauliflower resembles rice. Depending the size of your food processor, you will probably need to work in two or three batches. Or use a box grater and grate the cauliflower. Set aside.

2. Add the butter to a large skillet over medium-high heat. Add the garlic and cauliflower and stir to combine. Season with salt and pepper.

3. Cook the cauliflower mixture until the cauliflower just begins to soften, for about 4–5 minutes.

4. Remove from the heat, adjust the seasonings, and stir in the lemon juice and fresh herbs, if using.

PER SERVING (WITHOUT OPTIONAL INGREDIENTS): 145 calories, 5g protein, 10g total fat, 8g total carbohydrate

BROCCOLI RICE

Makes 2 servings

This recipe is a brilliant way to use up broccoli stalks. If you don't have a food processor, simply grate the broccoli on the coarsest side of a box grater.

> 4 uncooked broccoli stalks (the dried ends trimmed), cut into large chunks
>
> 1½ tablespoons butter
>
> 1–4 garlic cloves, minced
>
> Salt and pepper, to taste

1. Place the broccoli stalks in the bowl of a food processor and pulse until they resemble rice grains. Do not overprocess.

2. In a large sauté pan over medium heat, add the butter and garlic. Cook for 1–2 minutes, until the garlic is softened.

3. Add the broccoli rice, salt, and pepper, and cook just until tender, for about 8–10 minutes.

PER SERVING: 185 calories, 3g protein, 12g total fat, 6g total carbohydrate

SPIRALIZED VEGGIE PASTA

Makes 1 or 2 servings

This is a fun recipe if you have a spiralizer attachment for your stand mixer or food processor. You can also use a handheld version or—the easiest option—simply purchase a tub of already spiralized veggies in the produce section of your local grocery store.

> 1 peeled and trimmed root, bulb, or marrow vegetable, or 2–4 ounces spiralized vegetables
>
> 1 tablespoon butter or another fat (Bacon fat is nice.)
>
> Salt and pepper, to taste

1. Using a spiralizer attachment on your food processor or stand mixer, or a mechanical spiralizer or handheld spiralizer, spiralize one vegetable per serving. (Large vegetables, such as rutabagas and eggplants, will make 2 servings.) If using prepared spiralized vegetables, skip this step.

2. Place a large sauté pan over medium-high heat and add the butter. When it melts, add the spiralized veggie and

sauté for 5 minutes, stirring gently to coat all strands with butter.

3. Season with salt and pepper to taste.

4. Use in your favorite recipe or store in a covered container for up to two days in the refrigerator.

CALORIE, FAT, PROTEIN, AND CARBOHYDRATE COUNTS WILL VARY.

* Vegetables are important in your diet but can be carb-heavy. Stick to low-carb veggies such as jicama, white-fleshed sweet potato, turnip, rutabaga, kohlrabi, zucchini, or eggplant for this dish.

Serve spiralized zucchini noodles with Keto Meatballs (page 21) for the dish shown on the cover. If desired, you can add Versatile Marinara Sauce (page 26).

CAULIFLOWER MASH

Makes about 4 servings

I first tasted mashed cauliflower in a macrobiotic cooking class back in the early 2000s. It was seasoned with miso paste and caramelized onions, and it was fantastic! This version—without miso—is just as fantastic. Enjoy!

1 large head cauliflower, cut into florets

3 tablespoons butter

2 tablespoons cream

Salt and pepper, to taste

OPTIONAL: 1-2 teaspoons lemon juice, to keep the cauliflower white

OPTIONAL: 2 tablespoons fresh herbs, such as parsley or chives

1. Place a saucepan of salted water over high heat and bring to a boil Add the cauliflower and boil until fork-tender.

2. Transfer to a food processor and puree with butter, cream, salt, pepper, and lemon juice, if using. Process until smooth.

3. Adjust the seasoning and top with herbs, if using.

PER SERVING (WITHOUT OPTIONAL INGREDIENTS): 150 calories, 5g protein, 11g total fat, 8g total carbohydrate

CHEDDAR CAULIFLOWER MASH

Omit the lemon juice and herbs. Stir in 1½ cups shredded cheddar cheese before step 3.

BROCCOLI MASH

Makes 2 servings

This bright green dish looks nothing like mashed potatoes, but it has that same smooth, creamy texture. Use peeled leftover broccoli stalks, or fresh or frozen broccoli florets

2 cups broccoli florets and/or peeled stalks

1½ tablespoons butter

1 small garlic clove

Salt and pepper, to taste

OPTIONAL: 1 tablespoon fresh chives, parsley, basil, or other herb

1. Place a saucepan of salted water over high heat and bring to a boil. Add the broccoli and boil until fork-tender.

2. Remove the broccoli and while it is still warm, place it in the bowl of a food processor with the remaining ingredients and pulse until smooth.

3. Alternately, you could use an immersion blender to blend the remaining ingredients into the cooked broccoli.

4. Adjust the seasonings and serve immediately, or place in a covered container in the refrigerator for up to two days.

PER SERVING (WITHOUT OPTIONAL INGREDIENTS): 175 calories, 5g protein, 5g total fat, 5g total carbohydrate

THAI RED CURRY CHICKEN

If you don't have chicken, use pork. If you can't find red curry paste, use green. This recipe is more of a guide than a set of iron-clad culinary rules.

1 tablespoon coconut oil

1 onion, thinly sliced into half moons

1 ½ pounds boneless, skinless chicken thighs, chopped

2 cloves minced garlic

1 red bell pepper, sliced lengthwise

1 small zucchini, cut into half-moon slices

1 cup fresh mushrooms, sliced

1 can (14 ounces) coconut milk

3 tablespoons Thai red curry paste

½ tablespoon soy sauce

OPTIONAL: 2 tablespoons minced fresh cilantro, mint, or holy basil (or a combination)

Cauliflower Rice (page 111) or Broccoli Rice (page 112)

1. Add the oil to a large frying pan over medium-high heat. When warm, add the onions and sauté until just starting to soften.

2. Add the chicken and minced garlic. Cook until the chicken is nearly cooked through, about 5–7 minutes. Add the red pepper, zucchini, and mushrooms, and sauté just until the red peppers are tender-crisp.

3. Lower the heat to medium-low and stir in the coconut milk, red curry paste, and soy sauce, and simmer for 10 minutes or until thickened.

4. Stir in the herbs, if using, and remove from the heat.

5. Enjoy with Cauliflower Rice or Broccoli Rice.

PER SERVING (WITHOUT OPTIONAL INGREDIENTS): 410 calories, 23g protein, 30g total fat, 12g total carbohydrate

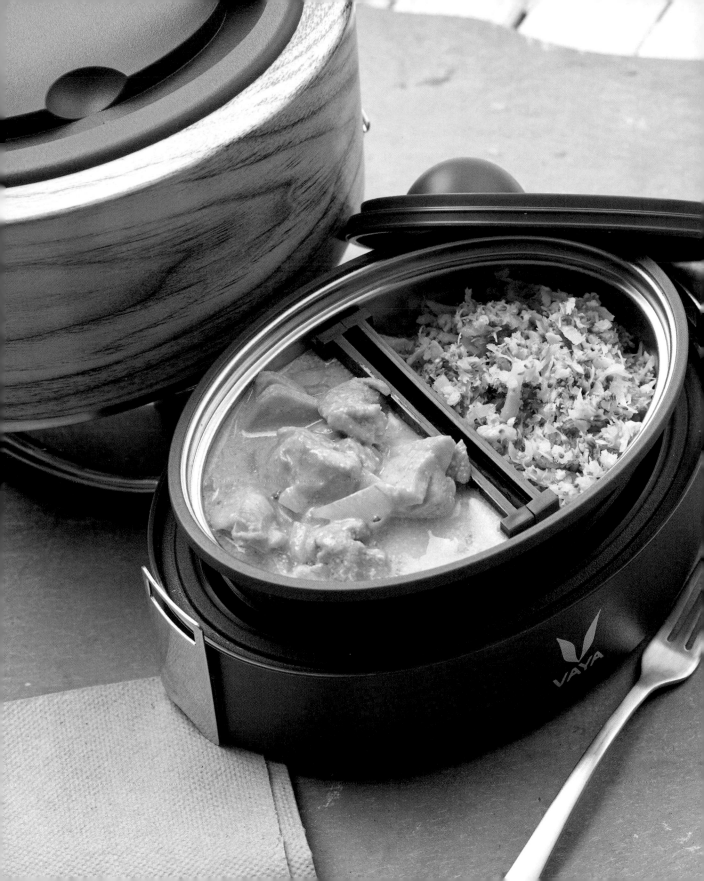

KETO INDI CURRY

Indian-style curries are the ultimate comfort foods, both soothing and exciting at the same time. Feel free to add a cup of greens (such as spinach) or another veggie to this recipe.

3 tablespoons coconut oil

1½ pounds boneless, skinless chicken thighs, chopped

1 tablespoon (or more) Madras-style curry powder

½ onion, chopped

2 garlic cloves, minced

1 (1-inch) slice of ginger, peeled and minced (or grated)

1 can (14 ounces) coconut milk

1 cup chicken broth

Salt and pepper, to taste

Broccoli Rice (page 112)

1. Add the oil to a large saucepan over medium-high heat.

2. Add the chicken and let brown for 5 minutes. Do not let the chicken cook completely.

3. Add the curry powder, onion, garlic, and ginger to the pan with the chicken and cook for 2 minutes.

4. Stir in the coconut milk and broth. Allow to simmer for 30-40 minutes, until slightly reduced and thickened.

5. Enjoy with Broccoli Rice.

PER SERVING: 350 calories, 26g protein, 29g total fat, 6g total carbohydrate

CREAMY FISH CASSEROLE

Makes 4 servings

This casserole, while reminiscent of Mom's tuna casseroles, is not only dressier, it's keto-friendly. If you don't have fish, use shrimp, chicken, or turkey. If you don't have broccoli, use asparagus, zucchini, or cauliflower.

1 tablespoon butter

½ pound of broccoli tops, separated into small florets

1 shallot, minced

1 tablespoon small capers

Salt and pepper, to taste

¾ pound whitefish, salmon, tuna, or another uncooked fish, cut into bite-size pieces

⅔ cup heavy cream

½ tablespoon Dijon mustard

2 teaspoons dried herb of choice, such as parsley, dill, or cilantro (or 2 tablespoons fresh)

1. Preheat the oven to 400°F.

2. Add the butter to a large frying pan over medium-high heat. Add the broccoli and shallot, and sauté until the broccoli is just barely tender, for about 5 minutes.

3. Add the capers, salt, and pepper, and sauté for 1 minute.

4. Transfer the sautéed vegetables to a casserole dish.

5. Gently stir the fish into the vegetables and set aside.

6. In a large bowl, whisk together the cream, mustard, herbs, salt, and pepper. Pour over the fish and vegetables.

7. Bake, uncovered, for 20 minutes, or until the fish is cooked through and flakes easily with a fork.

PER SERVING: 175 calories, 27g protein, 25g total fat, 8g total carbohydrate

PIZZA SPAGHETTI CASSEROLE

Makes 4 servings

Spaghetti squash gets its name from its stringy flesh, which resembles pasta. Yet, unlike pasta, spaghetti squash is gluten-free and great for keto eaters. Enjoy it in this meaty, pizza-like casserole.

1 pound ground beef,

1 pound bulk Italian sausage, sweet or hot

1 or 2 garlic cloves, minced

1 tablespoon dried oregano

½ tablespoon dried basil

Pinch of crushed red pepper flakes

Salt and pepper, to taste

1½ cups tomato puree

½ cup grated Parmesan cheese

1 (2-pound) spaghetti squash, cooked and flesh removed (see tip)

2 cups mozzarella cheese, divided

1. Place a large skillet over medium-high heat and add the ground beef, Italian sausage, garlic, oregano, basil, red pepper flakes, salt, and pepper. Cook until the meat is browned and no longer pink. Drain the grease, if desired.

2. Stir in the tomato puree and Parmesan and allow to cook until thickened, for about 10 minutes.

3. In the meantime, preheat the oven to 375°F.

4. Grease a casserole dish with a bit of coconut oil, avocado oil, olive oil, lard, or bacon fat. Add the cooked spaghetti squash to the bottom of the dish and sprinkle with salt and pepper to taste.

5. Layer 1½ cups of the mozzarella directly on top of the spaghetti squash.

6. Pour the meat mixture on top.

7. Top with the remaining ½ cup of mozzarella and bake until bubbly, for about 20 minutes.

8. Remove from the oven and let rest for at least 10 minutes before serving.

PER SERVING: 408 calories, 20g protein, 22g total fat, 6g total carb

How to cook spaghetti squash

If you've never cooked a spaghetti squash before, here is how I like to do it: Preheat the oven to 400°F. Slice the spaghetti squash in half down its length. Remove the seeds. Rub ½–1 tablespoon of your favorite oil or fat (such as bacon fat, lard, or butter) on the exposed interior flesh of the squash. Add salt and pepper to taste. If desired, add your favorite spices or dried herbs. Place the squash, cut side down, on an ungreased baking sheet. Bake for about 45 minutes, or until the vegetable is fork-tender. Remove from the oven, and allow to cool to room temperature. Using a fork, scrape out the spaghetti-like strands into a bowl. Use immediately or store in a covered container in your refrigerator for 2–3 days.

STUFFED CABBAGE ROLLS

Makes 6 servings

Cabbage rolls are easy, healthy, and versatile. You can use ground pork, turkey, or chicken in place of beef.

1 medium head cabbage (about 2 pounds)

1 pound ground beef

1 ½ cups Cauliflower Rice (page 111)

⅓ cup chopped fresh parsley

3 garlic cloves, minced

Salt and pepper, to taste

1 teaspoon sweet paprika

4 cups tomato sauce or Versatile Marinara Sauce (page 26)

1. Remove any dry or broken outer leaves from the cabbage head before coring it, being careful not to split the head or tear any of the leaves. Set aside.

2. Place a large pot of salted water over high heat and bring to a boil.

3. Lower the prepared cabbage head into the boiling water, making sure the entire head is submerged. Boil for 8–10 minutes, or until the head is softened, but not soft or soggy or mushy.

4. Place the cabbage in a colander in the sink and allow cold water to run over it to stop the cooking process. Let the cabbage head drain while you continue with the recipe.

5. In a large sauté pan, combine the beef, cauliflower rice, parsley, garlic, salt, pepper, and paprika. Cook over medium-high heat until the meat is browned.

6. Lightly grease a 9×12-inch baking dish with a bit of coconut oil, avocado oil, olive oil, lard, or bacon fat. Set aside.

7. Preheat the oven to 350°F.

8. Gently peel the outer 8 leaves from the prepared cabbage head to use for the cabbage rolls. With a sharp paring knife, shave off any thick ribs from the outside of the leaves.

9. Lay a cabbage leaf out in front of you, placing the base side at the bottom.

10. Place 2 tablespoons of the beef mixture about 2 inches above the bottom edge and roll. Place, seam-side down, in the prepared baking dish. Continue with the remaining 7 cabbage leaves.

11. Pour the tomato sauce over the cabbage rolls, cover dish with foil, and bake for 45–60 minutes, or until the rolls are tender.

12. Remove from the oven and let rest for 20 minutes before serving.

PER SERVING: 250 calories, 20g protein, 18g total fat, 8g total carbohydrate

KETO SHEPHERD'S PIE

Makes 6 servings

Shepherd's pie is a popular pub casserole featuring seasoned ground meat resting beneath a blanket of mashed potatoes. This yummy keto version replaces the carb-heavy potatoes with (you guessed it!) cauliflower.

1 pound ground lamb

1 pound ground beef

½ cup chopped onion

Salt and pepper, to taste

1 clove garlic, minced

½ cup dry red wine

2 tablespoons chopped fresh rosemary (or 2 teaspoons dried)

1 recipe Cheddar Cauliflower Mash (page 113)

1. Preheat the oven to 400°F.

2. In a large skillet over medium heat, brown the lamb and beef until cooked through, about 10–12 minutes. Using a slotted spoon, remove the meat to a separate plate or bowl. Drain the grease that has collected in the pan, leaving 1–2 tablespoons of oil behind in the pan. Return the pan to the heat and add the onion, salt, and pepper. Cook until the onion is translucent, for about 5 minutes. Add the garlic and cook until fragrant, 1 minute more.

3. Return the meat to the pan, and add the wine and rosemary. Cook until the wine is mostly evaporated and the juices have thickened, 4–5 minutes. Transfer the meat mixture to a 2-quart casserole dish

4. Spread the Cheddar Cauliflower Mash over the meat mixture in the casserole dish, and bake for 20 minutes or until bubbling and golden.

5. Allow casserole to sit for 10 minutes once removed from the oven.

PER SERVING: 290 calories, 21g protein, 20g total fat, 8g total carbohydrate

KETO ITALIANO LASAGNA

Makes 4 servings

This alternative lasagna uses kale leaves instead of sheets of pasta. If you can't eat kale—or just don't like it—you can use chard (just reduce the cooking time by half).

1 tablespoon extra-virgin olive oil

1 pound Italian sausage, sweet or hot, casings removed

2 medium bunches of kale, stems and ribs removed, roughly chopped

3 cups Versatile Marinara Sauce (page 26), divided

1 tablespoon fresh basil, minced (or 1 teaspoon dried)

Salt and pepper, to taste

¼ cup finely grated Parmesan cheese, divided

2 cups grated mozzarella cheese, divided

1. Preheat the oven to 375°F.

2. Prepare a 9×12-inch baking dish by rubbing it with olive oil. Set aside.

3. Place the oil in a large frying pan over medium-high heat. Add the sausage and cook until browned, breaking it up with a spoon.

4. Add the marinara sauce, basil, and salt and pepper to taste, and let simmer for about 20 minutes until slightly reduced.

5. While the sauce is cooking, place a large pot of salted water over high heat and bring to a vigorous boil. Add the kale and cook for 4 minutes, or just until bright and wilted. Be sure to not overcook.

6. Immediately drain the kale into a colander and allow cold water to run over the kale to stop the cooking process. Let the kale drain in the sink while you attend to the sauce. (You want the kale as dry as possible. If it still seems wet when you are ready to cook with it, lay it on paper towels to absorb excess water, or run it through a salad spinner.)

7. In the baking dish, layer half of the kale, half of the sauce, half of the Parmesan, and half of mozzarella.

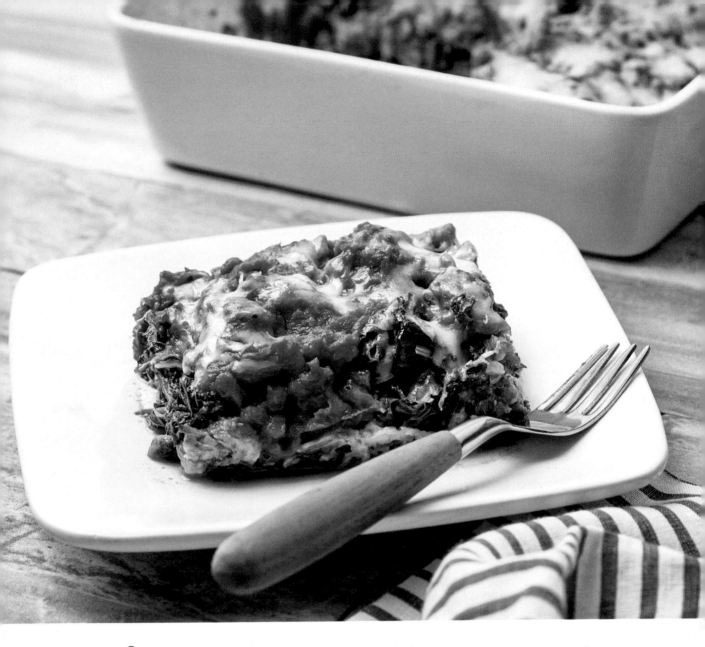

8. Repeat with another layer of the remaining kale, sauce, Parmesan, and mozzarella. Cover the dish with foil and bake for about 15 minutes, then remove the foil and bake for another 20 minutes, or until the casserole is bubbling and the cheese is starting to brown.

9. Let the lasagna sit for about 10 minutes before serving.

PER SERVING: 400 calories, 29g protein, 21g total fat, 15g total carb

CHAPTER SIX

KETO FAT BOMBS

If you're a dedicated keto eater, you know all about fat bombs. If you're new to this way of eating, however, let me define the term: Fat bombs are literally fat-infused finger foods you eat for a quick infusion of calories and fat. Many keto eaters use fat bombs as a late-morning or midafternoon snack; others add a fat bomb to their lunch to round out a lean microwaved convenience meal. The fat bombs in this chapter are yummy and filled with healthy fats—as well as plenty of antioxidants. Your body and taste buds will be happy.

SAVORY BOMBS

BACON-LIVERWURST BALLS

Makes about 12 balls

Liverwurst is high in iron and protein and has a nice amount of fat, which is why it's a keto staple. If you like Braunschweiger, you'll love this no-cook recipe!

8 ounces liverwurst, at room temperature

6 ounces cream cheese, softened

¼ cup chopped pecans

1–2 teaspoons mustard

Salt and pepper, to taste

8 slices crisp cooked bacon, finely chopped

1. Place the liverwurst, cream cheese, pecans, mustard, salt, and pepper in a food processor and pulse until just combined.

2. Using a small cookie scoop or large spoon, scoop out 12 portions and roll into balls.

3. Place the balls on a plate or baking sheet, and chill in the refrigerator for at least 30 minutes.

4. Roll each ball in bacon. Eat immediately or store in a covered container for up to a five days. Serve cold or at room temperature.

PER SERVING (ONE BALL): 147 calories, 8g protein, 13g total fat, 2g total carbohydrate

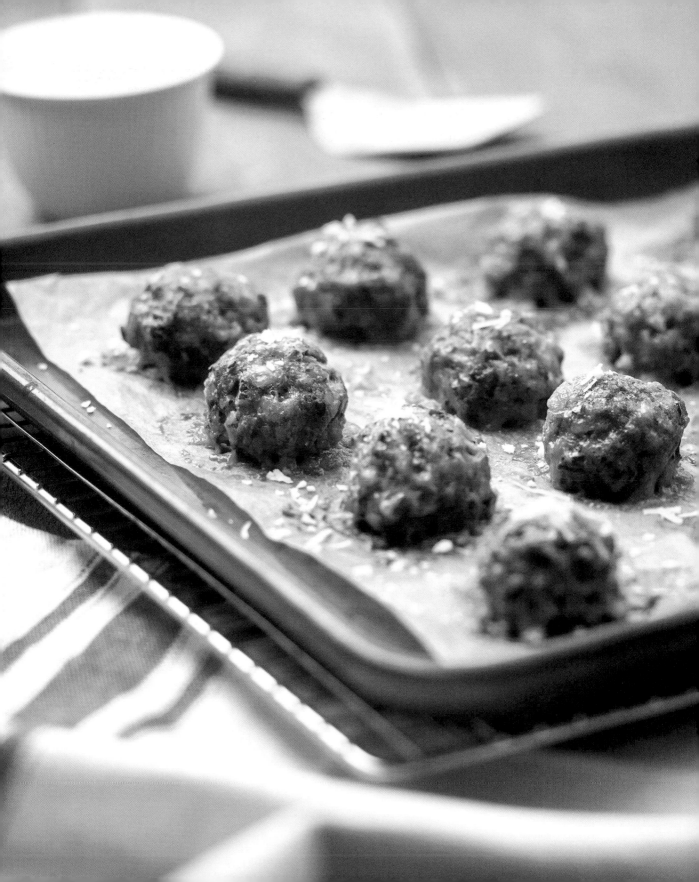

SAUSAGE PUFFS

These yummy puffs make a great appetizer at your next party. Buy bulk ground sausage, or buy links and remove the casings.

1 pound pork breakfast or Italian sausage, uncooked

1 egg

1 cup finely ground pecans, almonds, or nut of choice

8 ounces extra sharp cheddar cheese

¼ cup grated Parmesan cheese

1 tablespoon butter, coconut oil, lard, or another fat

2 teaspoons baking powder

Salt and pepper, to taste

1. Preheat the oven to 350°F.

2. Add all ingredients to the bowl of a stand mixer and mix on a low speed until completely combined. The sausage will be chunky.

3. Using a small cookie scoop or large spoon, scoop out 20 portions and roll into balls.

4. Place the balls on a cookie sheet lined with foil or parchment paper.

5. Bake for 16–20 minutes or until browned and just firm to the touch.

6. Eat immediately or store in the refrigerator for up to three days.

PER SERVING (ONE PUFF): 79 calories, 5g protein, 7g total fat, 1g total carbohydrate

MEATY JALAPEÑO POPPERS

This keto-friendly version of the beloved appetizer uses fresh peppers and cream cheese. If you have leftover meatloaf or meatballs (like Keto Meatballs page 21), or leftover bacon, you can crumble it up and substitute it for the ground meat, garlic, and spices, skipping step 2 and adding the leftover meat at step 3.

6 ounces ground beef, bison, chorizo, or another ground meat

1 garlic clove, minced

1 teaspoon cumin

1 teaspoon dried oregano

Salt and black pepper, to taste

8 medium jalapeños, cut in half and seeds removed

2 ounces cream cheese

1. Preheat the oven to 350°F and lightly grease a baking sheet with a bit of coconut oil, avocado oil, olive oil, lard, or bacon fat.

2. Add the meat, garlic, cumin, and oregano to a large pan over medium heat. Cook until browned, and season with salt and pepper. Set aside.

3. Smear each jalapeño half with cream cheese, leaving room for the meat mixture. Once it has cooled, spoon the cooked meat mixture into each prepared jalapeño half.

4. Place the poppers on a baking rack and bake for 30 minutes.

5. Eat immediately or store in the refrigerator for up to five days.

PER SERVING (ONE PEPPER): 144 calories, 8g protein, 5g total fat, 1g total carb

SALMON DAIRY BLOBS

This elegant recipe is a lovely way to get fish into your diet. It is ideal for brunch or even a dinner appetizer.

½ cup cream cheese

⅓ cup butter

8 ounces smoked salmon

1 tablespoon fresh lemon juice

1–2 tablespoons freshly chopped dill (or 1 teaspoon dried), plus more for garnish

Pinch of salt

1. Line a tray with parchment paper. Set aside.

2. Place all ingredients into a food processor. Pulse until smooth.

3. Using a cookie scoop or large spoon, create small fat bombs using about 2½ tablespoons of the mixture per portion. Garnish with more dill and place in the refrigerator for 1–2 hours or until firm.

4. Eat as-is or on top of crunchy lettuce leave, or enjoy as a spread on cucumber slices or with spears of endive or romaine lettuce. Store in the refrigerator for up to five days.

PER SERVING (ONE BLOB): 147 calories, 4g protein, 16g total fat, 1g total carbohydrate

* Instead of creating blobs, spoon the mixture into an airtight container. Eat immediately or store in the refrigerator for up to one week. Spoon out about 2½ tablespoons per serving.

PIZZA BOMBS

Pizza is one of the world's favorite foods, so there is a good chance that this may be one of your favorite fat bombs!

3 ½ ounces cream cheese

¼ cup butter, softened

1 tablespoon chopped fresh basil (or 1 teaspoon dried)

2 teaspoons chopped fresh oregano leaves (or 1 teaspoon dried)

¼ cup oil-packed sun-dried tomatoes, drained and chopped

¼ cup pitted Kalamata olives, chopped

2 cloves garlic, minced

Salt and pepper, to taste

¼ cup grated Parmesan cheese

1. Place all the ingredients in the bowl of a food processor and pulse a few times until just combined.

2. Chill the mixture in the refrigerator for 30 minutes, or until firm.

3. Using a small cookie scoop or large spoon, scoop out 8 portions and roll into balls.

4. Eat immediately or store in the refrigerator for up to five days.

PER SERVING (ONE BOMB): 163 calories, 4g protein, 17g total fat, 2g total carbohydrate

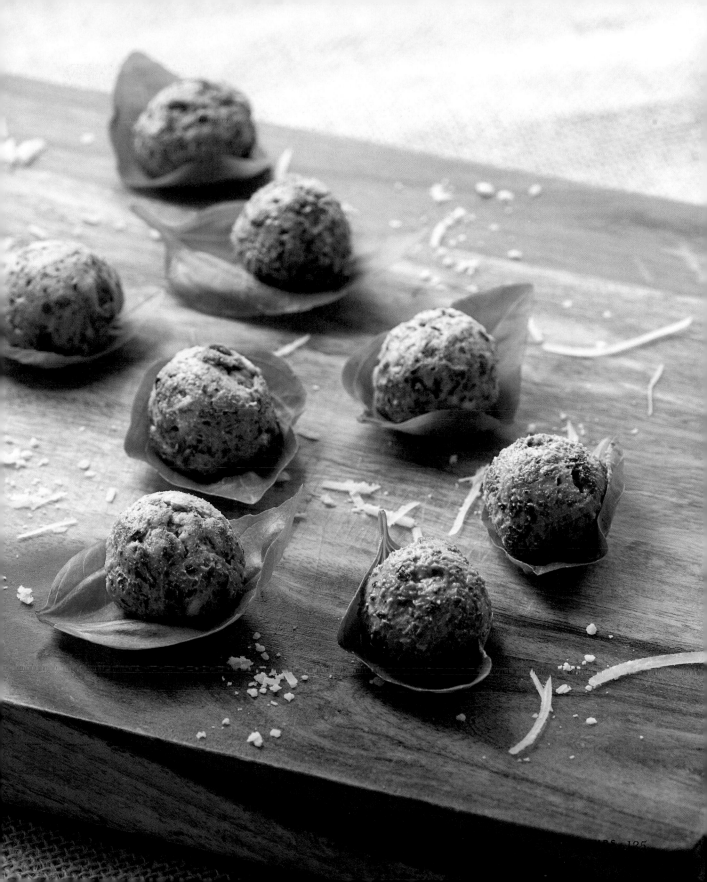

BACON AVOCADO PLOPS

Makes 6 plops

If you love bacon and avocado sandwiches as much as I do, you'll love these addictive goodies. Feel free to adjust the spiciness.

4 large slices bacon

½ large avocado, pit and peel removed

¼ cup coconut oil, room temperature

1 small chile pepper, minced

⅓ cup finely chopped onion

2 tablespoons freshly chopped cilantro

1 tablespoon fresh lime juice

¼ teaspoon salt or more, to taste

Black pepper, to taste

1. Preheat the oven to 375°F. Line a baking tray with parchment paper. Lay out the bacon strips, leaving space so they don't overlap. Place the tray in the oven and cook for about 10–15 minutes, until golden brown. Remove from the oven and set aside to cool.

2. Place the avocado, coconut oil, chile pepper, onion, cilantro, and lime juice into a bowl and season with salt and pepper. Mash with a potato masher or a fork until well combined.

3. Add the bacon grease from the tray on which you baked the bacon into the avocado mixture, and mix well. Cover with foil and place in the refrigerator for 20–30 minutes to firm up.

4. Crumble the bacon into small pieces and spread on a plate or baking tray.

5. Remove the guacamole mixture from the refrigerator and create 6 balls using an cookie scoop or large spoon. Roll each ball in the bacon crumbles, wrap and place on a tray. Eat immediately.

6. If not eating immediately, wrap each in plastic wrap and store in the refrigerator in an airtight container for up to five days.

PER SERVING (ONE PLOP): 156 calories, 4g protein, 15g total fat, 3g total carbohydrate

Fat Bombs 101

Fat bombs are mini meals, snacks, or treats that are high in fat and low in carbs and that you can enjoy as a quick breakfast (maybe paired with a green drink like Green Keto Lemonade page 161), eat as a quick midafternoon snack, use as a pre- or post-workout energizer, or munch on any time you need a hit of energy. Here are four facts about fat bombs:

1. **Ketogenic fat bombs are often small.** They are high in fat and often very filling, and come in the shape of balls, nuggets, patties, plops, or mini-muffins.

2. **Fat bombs can be savory or sweet.** What differentiates the sweeter fat bombs from conventional sugary treats is the sweetener. Because traditional sweeteners (think sugar, molasses, honey, apple juice concentrate) contain carbohydrates (a no-no on the ketogenic diet), stevia is used.

   FUN FACT: Stevia causes fewer stomach problems than sugar alcohols and culinary glycerins, which are often used in mainstream low-carb treats.

3. **Fat bombs contain a ton of healthy fats.** On a ketogenic diet (and kindred diets, such Atkins, South Beach, and paleo) eating healthy fat is highly important to lower inflammation in your body. Most fat bombs contain coconut oil, coconut butter, cacao butter, and/or avocado for this reason—plus these ingredients are solid at cooler temperatures and therefore act, as a binder in most fat bomb recipes. They often last five days (or up to a week or more if it's a sweet chocolate bomb) in the refrigerator in an airtight container.

4. **Fat bombs often contain nuts and seeds.** Many keto dieters avoid consuming too many nuts and seeds because they tend to be high in carbs and if heated can easily become oxidized. That being said, nuts and seeds add wonderful texture, healthy fats, and flavor to many fat bombs, so they are used sparingly.

SWEET BOMBS

MATCHA AND COCONUT FAT BALLS

Makes about 32 balls

Containing antioxidant-rich matcha, this rich, healthy, delicious treat is just different enough to catch your attention. Sometimes I like to add ⅛ teaspoon of ground star anise, or cardamom.

1 cup firm coconut oil (refrigerate to harden, if necessary)

1 cup creamy coconut butter, room temperature

½ cup coconut cream, refrigerated overnight

1 tablespoon + ½ teaspoon matcha green tea powder, divided

¼ teaspoon ground ginger

¼ teaspoon salt

1 teaspoon pure vanilla extract

1 cup finely shredded unsweetened coconut

1. In the bowl of a stand mixer fitted with a paddle attachment, add the coconut oil, coconut butter, coconut milk, ½ teaspoon of the matcha green tea powder, ginger, salt, and vanilla extract.

2. Mix on high speed until light and fluffy. Remove the bowl from the mixer and stash in the refrigerator for 1 hour or more to firm up.

3. While the mixture is firming up, whisk together the shredded coconut and the remaining 1 tablespoon of matcha powder in a large mixing bowl. Set aside.

4. Remove the mixture from the refrigerator. Using a small cookie scoop or large spoon, form 32 little balls, roughly the size of a gum ball.

5. Roll the balls quickly between the palms of your hands to smooth them into perfect balls. Then drop each ball into the bowl with the coconut-matcha mixture. Roll gently until completely coated.

6. Transfer your finished fat balls to an airtight container and keep refrigerated for up to ten days.

7. These can be eaten straight out of the refrigerator. but they are even better when you let them sit at room temperature for 10–15 minutes before to eating them.

PER SERVING (ONE BALL): 130 calories, 1g protein, 13g total fat, 2g total carbohydrate

* For this recipe, it's importance that the coconut oil and coconut cream be firm. Refrigerate both for at least 2 hours before you begin.

WHITE CHOCOLATE BOMBS

Makes about 12 balls

White chocolate is a creamy, fatty, thoroughly addictive substance. Personalize this recipe with spices, extracts, or add-ins like dried coconut, chocolate chips, or nuts.

¼ cup cocoa butter

¼ cup coconut oil

¼ finely shredded unsweetened coconut

10 drops liquid stevia

½ teaspoon vanilla extract

1. In the bowl of a double boiler set over low heat, melt together the cocoa butter and coconut oil.

2. Remove from the heat and stir in the shredded coconut, stevia, and vanilla extract.

3. Pour into molds or mini muffin cups.

4. Chill until hardened.

5. Remove from the molds. Eat immediately or store in a covered container in the refrigerator for up to 10 days.

PER SERVING (ONE BOMB): 128 calories, 1g protein, 11g total fat, 2g total carbohydrate

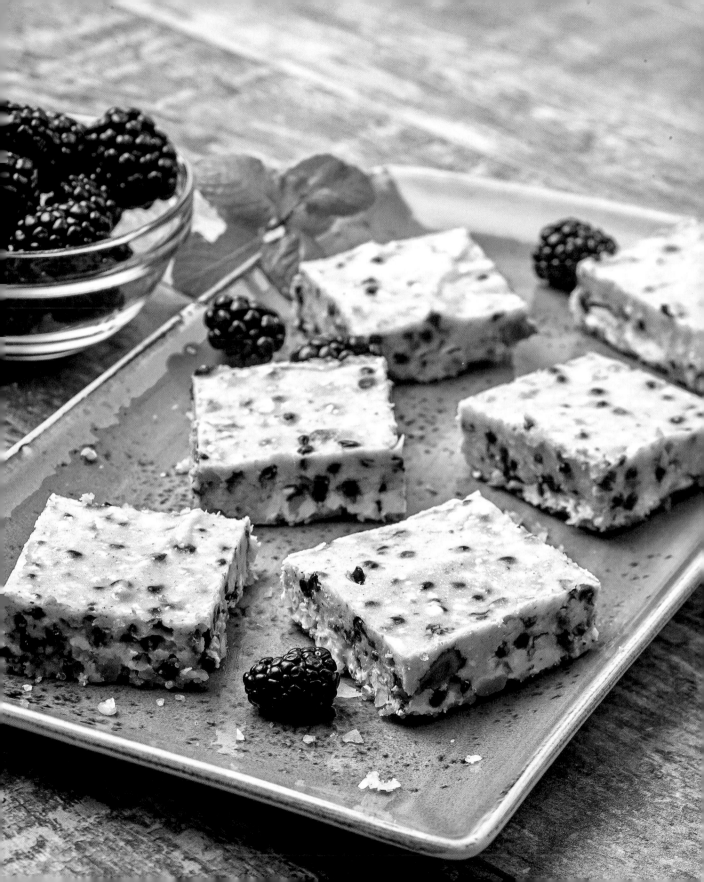

BLACKBERRY-NUT FAT SQUARES

Try this with raspberries for a more tart, pink fat bomb.

2 ounces ground macadamia nuts cashews, pistachios or another nut or mixture of nuts.

3 ½ ounces cream cheese, at room temperature

1 cup blackberries

¼ cup mascarpone cheese

½ cup butter

½ cup coconut oil

1 cup coconut butter

1 teaspsoon lime juice

Stevia, to taste

1. Preheat the oven to 325°F.

2. Press the ground nuts into the bottom of an 8-inch baking pan. Bake 5–7 minutes or until golden brown.

3. Remove from the oven and allow to cool slightly.

4. Spread the cream cheese over the nut crust.

5. In the bowl of a standing mixer set to low, mix together the blackberries, mascarpone cheese, butter, coconut oil, coconut butter, lime juice, and stevia until smooth.

6. Smooth the mixture over the cream cheese layer. Freeze for 30–60 minutes. Remove and eat immediately or store covered in the refrigerator for up to 10 days.

PER SERVING (ONE SQUARE): 390 calories, 5g protein, 45g total fat, 2 g total carbohydrate

* You can use a food processor or a coffee grinder for the nut crust.

ALMOND PISTACHIO SQUARES

Makes 36 squares

Nuts are used sparingly in keto recipes. Here, a sprinkling of pistachios (or another nuts) provide texture and flavor. You will adore these!

1 cup all-natural almond butter

1 cup coconut butter

1 cup coconut oil, chilled until semisolid

½ cup coconut cream, chilled overnight

¼ cup liquid coconut oil, pistachio oil, or ghee

1 teaspoon pure almond extract

2 teaspoons apple pie spice blend, chai spice blend, or pumpkin pie spice blend

¼ teaspoon salt

½ cup cacao butter, chopped and melted

¼ cup chopped pistachios, almonds, macadamia nuts, or walnuts

1. Grease and line a 9-inch square baking pan with foil or parchment paper, leaving 2 inches hanging on either side for easy unmolding. Set aside.

2. Add the almond butter, coconut butter, semisolid coconut oil, coconut cream, liquid oil, almond extract, spice blend, and salt to the bowl of a large stand mixer. Mix on low speed for 30 seconds to incorporate the ingredients.

3. Switch the mixer speed to high and mix until the mixture becomes airy and lighter in color, for about 3 minutes.

4. Reduce the mixer speed to low and slowly pour in the melted cacao butter. Mix for about 1 minute, or until well blended.

5. Transfer the mixture to the prepared pan and spread as evenly as possible. Press the chopped nuts into the top of the mixture.

6. Refrigerate for 4 hours, or until firm.

7. Cut into 36 squares.

8. Eat immediately or store in covered in the refrigerator for up to ten days.

PER SERVING (ONE SQUARE): 170 calories, 3g protein, 17g total fat, 3g total carbohydrate

SIMPLE NUT BUTTER FUDGE

Makes 12 pieces

This yummy treat is made with nut butter and coconut oil. Change things up by adding your favorite spices or extracts.

1 cup unsweetened peanut butter, almond butter, or another nut or seed butter of choice

1 cup coconut oil

¼ cup unsweetened coconut milk, coconut cream, dairy cream, or almond milk

OPTIONAL: Pinch of salt, only if needed

OPTIONAL: Dash of vanilla extract, or a sprinkle of cinnamon or nutmeg

OPTIONAL: 1–2 teaspoons liquid stevia

OPTIONAL: Unsweetened shredded coconut

1. Slightly melt or soften the peanut butter and coconut oil together in a small pot over low heat or in the microwave.

2. Add the warm mixture, along with all remaining ingredients except the shredded coconut, to the bowl of a food processor or stand mixer and process until combined and smooth.

3. Pour into the paper cups of a mini-muffin tray. Sprinkle a pinch of shredded coconut on each serving.

4. Refrigerate until set, for about 2 hours. Eat immediately or store in a covered container in the refrigerator for up to ten days.

PER SERVING (ONE PIECE, WITHOUT OPTIONAL INGREDIENTS): 156 calories, 4g protein, 30g total fat, 4g total carbohydrate

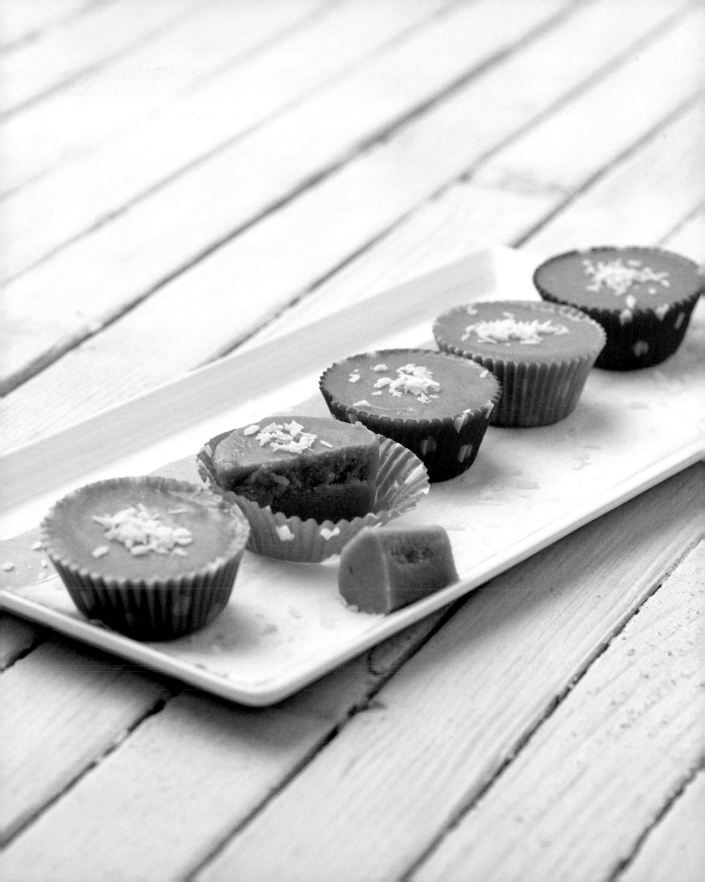

ORANGE-SCENTED CHOCOLATES

If you are also an orange chocolate fan, you will adore these fatabulous chocolates. If you're not as excited by the citrus-cocoa pairing, simply leave out the orange peel.

4 to 5 ounces of dark chocolate, 85% cocoa

¼ cup coconut oil

½–1 tablespoon finely chopped fresh orange peel (just the orange part)

OPTIONAL: ½ teaspoon or more vanilla extract

OPTIONAL: 10–15 drops of stevia

1 cup finely chopped pecans

1. Melt the chocolate in a double boiler over low heat.

2. Stir in coconut oil and, if using, vanilla extract and stevia.

3. Add the fresh orange peel.

4. Add the pecans and stir until coated.

5. Spoon the mixture into paper mini muffin or candy cups.

6. Place in the refrigerator for a couple of hours or until solid. Store in a covered container in the refrigerator or at room temperature, for up to 10 days.

PER SERVING (ONE CHOCOLATE): 88 calories, 3g protein, 8g total fat, 3g total carbohydrate

DIY Sweet Bomb Blueprint

If you have a blueprint, you can make anything your own, using what you have on hand. Yummy sweet fat bombs are no exception. Use this easy blueprint to come up with endless combinations of yummy, healthy, fatabulous bombs. Try it!

1 cup fat, or a mixture of two or three fats. These can include coconut oil, coconut cream, coconut butter, cocoa butter, avocado oil, avocado, ghee, butter, heavy cream, cream cheese, sour cream, or nut butter.

1 tablespoon or more flavoring. If making sweet bombs, this most often means dark chocolate, but it can also be a teaspoon of vanilla extract, spices, a few drops of peppermint extract, or the like.

2 tablespoons to ¼ cup texture-giving, "bulkifying" ingredients, such as shredded coconut, chia, cacao nibs, nuts, or seeds

1. Add all ingredients to a large bowl. Whisk together until thoroughly blended. If it makes sense to use a food processor or blender, do so, pulsing the ingredients together until blended.

2. Pour the mixture into small cups or molds. I like to use mini muffin cups.

3. Freeze or refrigerate until solid.

4. Store in a cool place or refrigerate for up to 10 days.

NOTE: If using nuts or seeds, less is more. These ingredients are best used in small amounts because they tend to be high in carbohydrates.

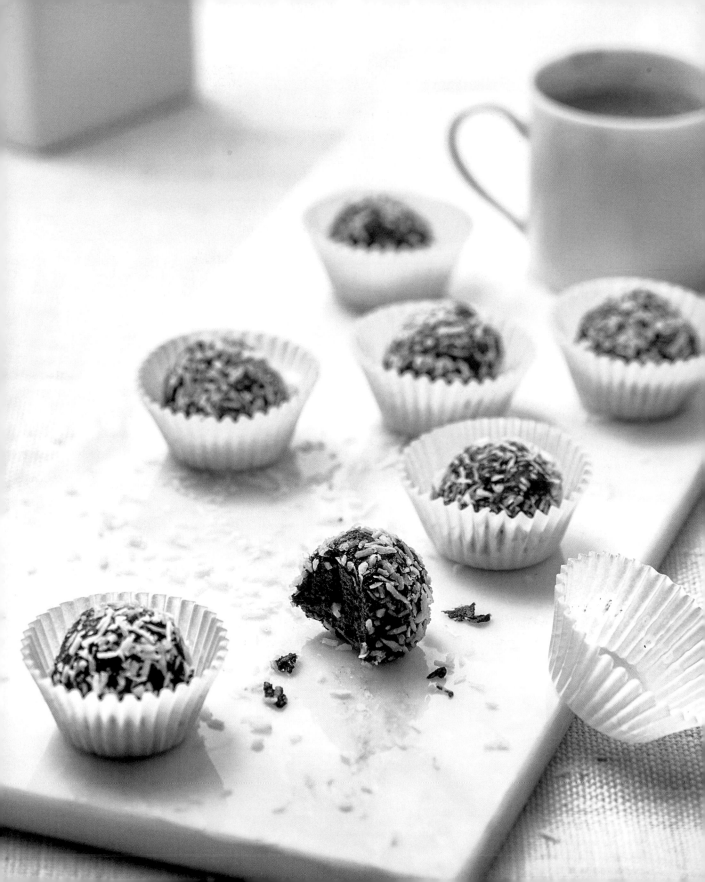

COCOA-COCONUT BALLS

Have some powdered peanut butter on hand that you don't know what to do with? Use it to make this recipe. If you can find it, powdered almond butter also works.

½ cup coconut oil

¼ cup finely chopped dark chocolate

¼ cup peanut butter powder

6 tablespoons shelled hemp seeds

2 tablespoons heavy cream or coconut cream

1 teaspoon vanilla extract

15–28 drops liquid stevia, or to taste

¼ cup unsweetened shredded coconut

1. In the bowl of a stand mixer or food processor, place the coconut oil, dark chocolate, peanut butter powder, and hemp seeds, and process until it forms a paste.

2. Add the heavy cream, vanilla, and stevia, and process until everything is combined and smooth. Store in the refrigerator for 30 minutes or more to chill.

3. Place the coconut on a plate or tray.

4. Using a small cookie scoop or large spoon, scoop out 12 portions and roll into balls.

5. Roll each ball into the coconut to coat. Eat immediately or store in a covered container in the refrigerator or freezer for up to ten days.

PER SERVING (ONE BALL): 190 calories, 5g protein, 19g total fat, 4g total carbohydrate

CHAPTER SEVEN

KETO DRINKS

When it comes to lunch, one of the most challenging questions for many keto eaters isn't "What can I eat?" It's "What can I drink?" Water is always a great lunchtime option, but what about those times when you want something fruity or are craving caffeine? These keto-approved sippers are easy, yummy, and portable—simply mix them up at home, pour them into a travel cup or vacuum bottle, and tuck them into your bag for a desk-side pick-me-up.

KETO COFFEE LATTE

Keto coffee—aka "bulletproof coffee"—is coffee that's been blended with fat. This lovely version can be made at home and warmed at the office for a late morning or early afternoon treat.

2 cups warm coffee of your choice, brewed as you normally would brew your coffee

2 tablespoons unsalted butter, preferably grass-fed

2 tablespoons organic coconut oil

OPTIONAL: 1 or more tablespoons coconut cream or heavy whipping cream

OPTIONAL: 1 teaspoon vanilla extract

Add all ingredients to a blender. Process until smooth and frothy.

PER SERVING (WITHOUT OPTIONAL INGREDIENTS): 220 calories, 1g protein, 26 g total fat, 0g total carbohydrate

ICED KETO COFFEE

This strong iced java drink is made keto-friendly with the addition of coconut oil and coconut cream.

12 ounces coffee of your choice, cooled

2 tablespoons organic coconut oil

2 tablespoons coconut cream or whipping cream

Add all ingredients to a blender. Process until smooth and frothy.

PER SERVING (WITH COCONUT CREAM): 124 calories, 1g protein, 18g total fat, 0g total carbohydrate

BULLETPROOF COFFEE DROPS

Makes 9 drops

These handy fat drops can be kept in your refrigerator and added to hot coffee, hot tea, or hot chocolate— or even tossed into a blender when making a smoothie. Plus, they can turn almost anything into a fat bomb!

½ cup ghee

1 cup organic coconut oil, melted

½ teaspoon cinnamon powder

¼ teaspoon sea salt

1. Combine all ingredients.

2. Whisk and pour into nine ice cube tray depressions, filling them to the top (or fill all twelve depressions in a standard ice cube tray partway). Place the tray in the freezer.

3. Once the drops have set, pop the drops from the tray into a glass container and cover. Store in the refrigerator until you are ready to use.

PER SERVING: 307 calories, 1g protein, 35g total fat, 0g total carbohydrate

* To make bulletproof coffee: Place one of the cubes and 10 ounces of hot coffee of your choice in a blender. Blend until well combined and foamy.

What is Ghee

* Ghee is a bit more than melted butter: It's a type of clarified butter that has been relieved of its milk solids and water. Ghee can be kept at room temperature and stays liquid when refrigerated. To make your own ghee, start with 1 pound of unsalted organic butter. Cut the butter into chunks and place in a small saucepan over medium heat. Once the butter is melted, reduce the heat to medium-low and allow to simmer for about 10–12 minutes. Remove the pan from the heat and skim away the foam that has developed on the top. Return the pan to the heat and allow the butter to simmer again. More foam will appear, and you may notice dark milk solids at the bottom of the pan. The butter will have become quite golden in color. Fully remove this foam, turn off the heat, and allow the butter to cool for 3 minutes. Pour the liquid butter through a fine sieve or strainer into a clean glass jar with a tightly fitting lid. Store at room temperature for up to 1 month or in the refrigerator for up to three months.

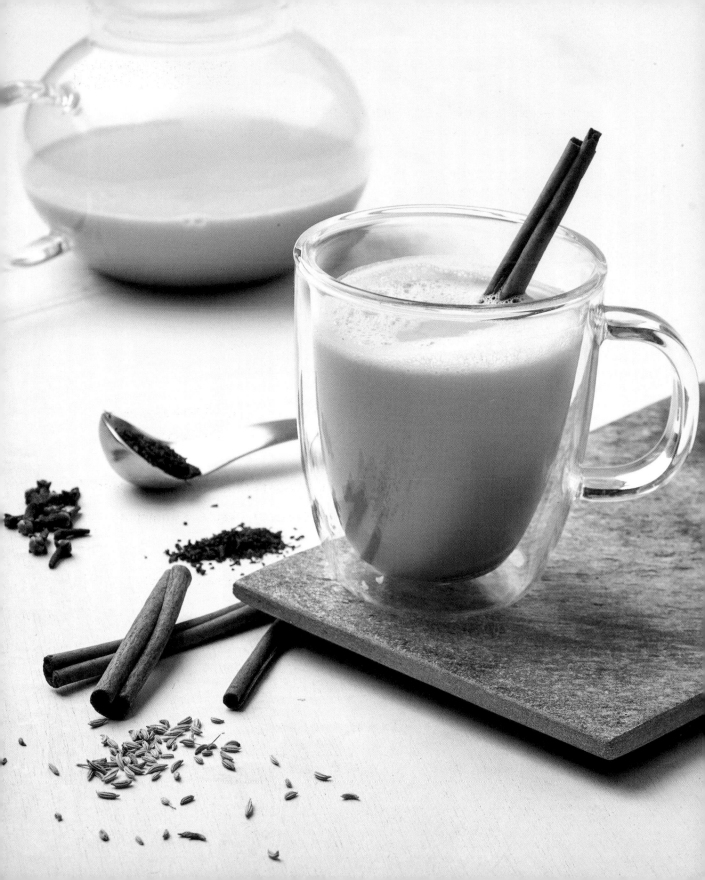

FATTY CHAI LATTE

Chai latte is one of my favorite warm drinks. This version tastes a lot like a drink at my favorite curry house. Yum!

½ teaspoon ground cinnamon

¼ teaspoon powdered ginger (or 1 teaspoon freshly grated)

¼ teaspoon ground allspice

¼ teaspoon whole fennel seeds

¼ teaspoon ground nutmeg

¼ teaspoon ground cloves

4 white cardamom pods

2 teaspoons vanilla extract

2 black tea bags

½ tablespoon coconut oil

1 cup coconut milk

1. In a small pot over medium heat, add 2–3 cups of water. Add the cinnamon, ginger, allspice, fennel, nutmeg, cloves, cardamom, and vanilla extract. Heat until the water boils.

2. Turn heat to the low, add the tea bags, and allow them to steep for 10 minutes.

3. Remove the tea bags and strain the liquid. Return the liquid to the pot and whisk in the coconut oil and coconut milk.

PER SERVING: 220 calories, 3g protein, 25g total fat, 3g total carbohydrate

ICED KETO TEA

If you've never made your own iced tea before, give it a try. It's fun; it's economical; it's quick; it's easy—and making your own iced tea ensures that you can use whatever kind of tea you'd like.

2-4 bags black, green, or white tea

3 cups boiling water

2 tablespoons unsalted butter

2 tablespoons coconut oil

¼ cup coconut milk, coconut cream, or heavy cream

1. Place the teabags in a pot or a heatproof bowl and pour the boiling water over them. Let the teabags steep in the water for 2–4 minutes, depending on how strong you like your tea.

2. Remove the teabags from the water.

3. Add the butter and coconut oil into the tea and whisk to blend.

4. Place the tea mixture in the fridge for to cool.

5. Add the coconut milk to the cooled tea and serve.

PER SERVING (WITH COCONUT MILK): 130 calories, 2g protein, 10g total fat, 2g total carbohydrate

Keto-Friendly Herbal Teas

Herbal teas—iced or hot—are fantastic, healthy, soothing drinks. But if you're a keto eater, be aware: fruit-flavored teas and teas that include pieces of dried fruit or fruit peel can contain sneaky carbohydrates. If you love herbal tea, stick to leaf-based infusions, such as peppermint.

KETO COCOA

Hot chocolate is a favorite afternoon office treat. For most people, however, their cocoa fix comes from an envelope. You can do so much better by whipping this up at home and bringing it with you to work in a vacuum bottle.

1 cup coconut milk

1 ounce unsalted butter, preferably grass-fed

½ tablespoon coconut oil

1 tablespoon cocoa powder

¼ teaspoon vanilla extract

OPTIONAL: Liquid stevia, to taste

1. In a small pot over medium heat, warm the coconut milk, butter, and coconut oil until the mixture begins to simmer.

2. Pour the liquid into a blender, and add the cocoa powder and vanilla extract. Process until blended and frothy.

3. Add stevia, if using, to taste.

PER SERVING: 220 calories, 5g protein, 35g total fat, 5g total carbohydrate

KETO COCOA SHAKE

Makes 2 servings

Smooth and creamy, this superfood smoothie will remind you of a milkshake, but it's better, thanks to a host of protein-rich, healthy fats.

1 tablespoon chia seeds

3 tablespoons water

1–1 ¼ cups full-fat coconut milk

½ small or medium avocado

1 tablespoon nut butter of choice

1 tablespoon cocoa powder

1 tablespoon coconut oil

1. In a small bowl, combine the chia seeds and 3 tablespoons of water. Soak for 10 minutes. You probably will have no remaining liquid at the end of 10 minutes, but if you do, go ahead and use it.

2. Place the chia seeds (and any remaining liquid, if there happens to be any) and all remaining ingredients in a blender and process until smooth. Add water, if you'd like a thinner shake.

PER SERVING: 400 calories, 6g protein, 39g total fat, 6g total carbohydrate

GREEN KETO LEMONADE

This tart, refreshing cooler is popular with my crowd, who all loves the refreshing taste of lemons. Substitute lime juice—or even the juice of Meyer lemons—if that's what you have.

Juice of 2 lemons

1 cup organic spinach

15 drops stevia extract, or to taste

1. Place all ingredients along with 2 $\frac{1}{2}$ cups of water in a high-powered blender.
2. Process until completely blended.

PER SERVING: 18 calories, 1g protein, 0g total fat, 5g total carbohydrate

CHIA-BERRY FRESCA

Makes 2 servings

This refreshing cooler features low-carb raspberries and the healthy fat, fiber, and protein of chia seeds.

2 tablespoons chia seeds

¼ cup water

1¾ cups coconut water

¼ cups frozen raspberries

1 tablespoon lemon or lime juice

OPTIONAL: Liquid stevia, to taste

1. Soak the chia seeds in ¼ cup of water for 10 minutes. You probably will have no remaining liquid at the end of 10 minutes, but if you do, go ahead and use it.

2. Place the chia seeds (and remaining liquid, if there happens to be any), coconut water, raspberries, and lemon juice in a blender and process until smooth.

3. Add liquid stevia, if using, to taste.

PER SERVING: 65 calories, 3g protein, 3g total fat, 6g total carbohydrate

Separation Anxiety

One complaint keto eaters often have about creamy drinks is that the fat often separates from the rest of the liquid. While this is not completely unavoidable, there are a few things you can do to keep the drink blended:

* Use frozen or cold ingredients when making drinks.

* Mix drinks using a high-powered blender, and puree the ingredients for at least 2 minutes.

* If you won't be enjoying your drink right away, store it in the refrigerator in a jar or similar container, and shake vigorously before enjoying.

BERRY CREAM SMOOTHIE

This luscious smoothie is filling enough to be a meal, especially when enjoyed with a cup of soup or a salad.

½ cup frozen strawberries or raspberries

¼ cup frozen blackberries

½ cup plain whole milk Greek yogurt

10 drops liquid stevia extract, or to taste

1 cup unsweetened coconut milk

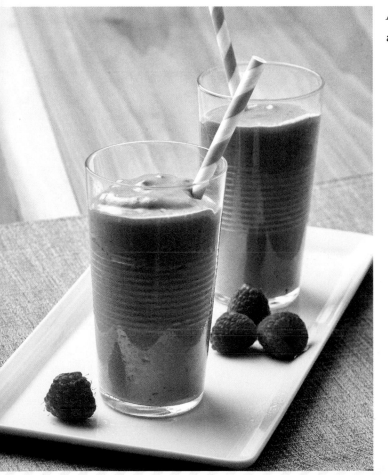

Add all ingredients to the blender and puree until smooth.

PER SERVING: 350 calories, 5g protein, 30g total fat, 7g total carbohydrate

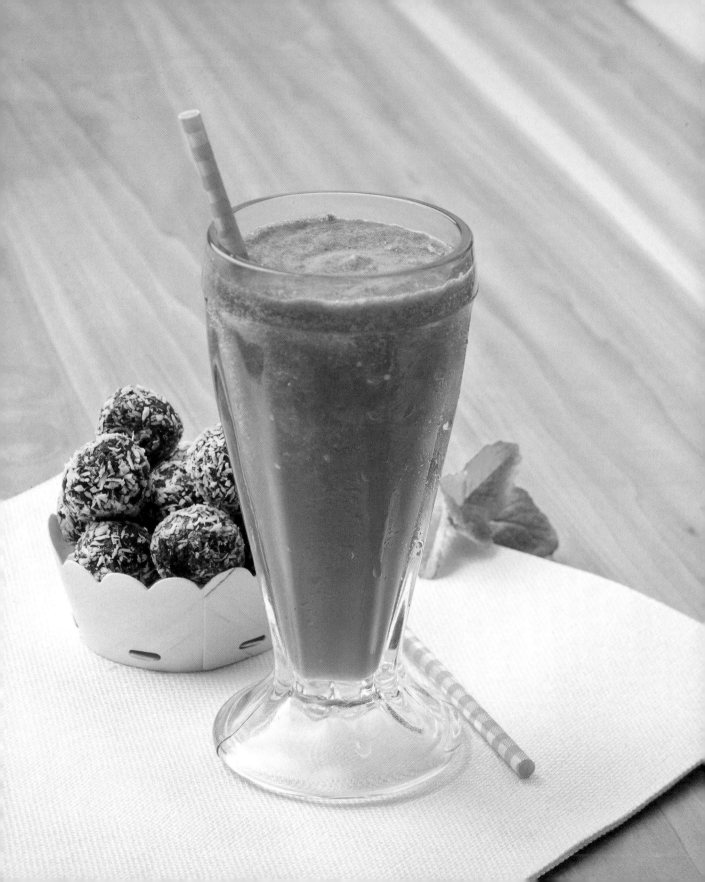

WATERMELON COOLER

If you're one of the many keto eaters who desperately miss fruit, this yummy cooler is for you. It's made with low-carb watermelon and is super-refreshing.

1½ pounds seedless watermelon cubes

½ cup coconut water

Juice of 1 lime

Pinch sea salt

1. Place all ingredients in a blender.
2. Process until smooth.

PER SERVING: 30 calories, 1g protein, 0g total fat, 4g total carbohydrate

* Wash down a Cocoa-Coconut Ball (page 151) with this refreshing drink.

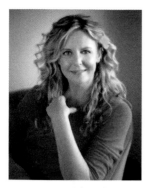

ABOUT THE AUTHOR

Stephanie Pedersen, CHHC, AADP, is a nutrition educator, cookbook author, and media host. Author of more than twenty books, Stephanie has a reputation for giving her private and corporate clients the edge they need to get whatever they want from life. She does this by helping individuals to lose weight, manage food allergies, and detoxify naturally, using food and lifestyle changes.

As Stephanie says, "I want health for everyone! I have seen firsthand with myself and my own clients that when one works to get clean and fit and address one's health challenges, life gets bigger. Life becomes outrageously fun and easy. You move healthfully through life with ease."

According to Stephanie, getting healthy doesn't have to be complicated or time-consuming. "As a mother, writer, nutrition educator, stagemom, and someone who loves to have time alone to wander local farmers' markets, I know that complicated, overly fussy diets, or an unnatural obsession with calorie-counting, are not the answers to getting and staying healthy." Instead, Stephanie espouses a life of love, laughter, daily exercise, and your favorite whole foods.

"We're lucky that we live in a time when more and more gorgeous whole food ingredients, organic produce, and humanely farmed meat are available. Let's celebrate our good fortune by exploring our many food and fitness options and experimenting with abandon."

You can find Stephanie online at www.StephaniePedersen.com, where you can read more about how she creates her own brand of healthy living. You'll find recipes, photos, tutorials, strategies, and more for creating a sane, productive, comfort-filled life. You can also access episodes of Stephanie's radio shows and podcasts, read chapters of her cookbooks, and offer feedback. Also by Stephanie Pedersen and Sterling Publishing:

Roots: The Complete Guide to the Underground Superfood

Berries: The Complete Guide to Cooking with Power-Packed Berriese

Coconut: The Complete Guide to the World's Most Versatile Superfood

The 7-Day Superfood Cleanse

Kale: The Complete Guide to the World's Most Powerful Superfood

ACKNOWLEDGMENTS

I couldn't have finished *Keto Lunches* without the support of my husband, Richard Joseph Demler, and our sons Leif Christian Pedersen, Anders Gyldenvalde Pedersen, and Axel SuneLund Pedersen. Thanks to my amazing clients for the constant inspiration you bring. Every day I am amazed at your drive, courage, and will. Getting healthy can be scary, and yet you see the joy in feeling your best, dive in, and create vibrant wellness for yourself. Yay, you! I am in awe of each of you.

Index